BELLYTALK

BELLY TALK

OTHER BOOKS BY JOHN SELBY

Therapeutic Massage
Visionetics
Powerpoint
Responsive Breathing
The See Clearly Book
The Visual Handbook
Finding Each Other
Immune-System Activation
Secrets of a Good Night's Sleep

JOHN SELBY

BELLYTALK

The New Body Book For Men

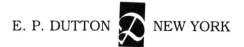

E. P. DUTTON · NEW YORK

Published in the United States by E. P. Dutton,
a division of Penguin Books USA Inc.,
2 Park Avenue, New York, N.Y. 10016.

Library of Congress Cataloging-in-Publication Data
Selby, John.
    Bellytalk: the new body book for men / John Selby. — 1st ed.
        p.   cm.
    ISBN 0-525-48526-0
    1. Men—Health and hygiene.   2. Abdomen.   3. Exercise for
men. 4. Physical fitness for men.   I. Title.
    RA777.8.S47   1990
    613.7'0449—dc20   89-36337
                                                                  CIP

Designed by Margo D. Barooshian

10 9 8 7 6 5 4 3 2 1

First Edition

Contents

Introduction: Men Growing Up and Out   1

1   Muscletalk   9

2   A Conversation with Your Belly   19

3   Remembering Slimmer Days   27

4   Self-Image Alterations   35

5   Your Warrior Spirit   51

6   On Men Counting Calories   58

7   Flat-Belly Movement Routines   68

8   Emotional and Sexual Considerations   81

9   Discipline Versus Self-Love   93

10   Wisdom of the Belly   100

11   Machines That Help   107

12   Belly Consciousness   114

Final Words/A Lifetime Fitness Plan   119

Supporting Cassette Programs   128

BELLYTALK

Introduction:
Men Growing Up and Out

This book is going to look intimately at one of those timeless and universal conditions that men everywhere either learn to accept and live with, or struggle to change for the better. Whether short or tall, rich or poor, gay or straight, black or white or whatever color you choose, men, as they mature toward middle age, have always been challenged by the threat or the accomplished fact of an overgrown midriff, an extended waistline, a protruding belly.

The laughing Buddha, it should be pointed out, was a great hero in ancient times who was portrayed in statues as having quite a large belly. In many ways, and in many cultures, a big belly has been considered a positive emblem of happiness, success, and even enlightened awareness.

But these days most of us do not see a big belly in quite this positive a light. We are afraid that a big belly, or even one that is beginning slightly to overgrow its confines, is a symbol of a loss of youthful strength and attractiveness. We are also embarrassed that a bulging midriff might indicate a lack of discipline in both our exercising and our eating habits. And we are certainly worried that our extra pounds and stuffed intestines may lead to eventual health problems if we don't do something about them.

I should admit right at the beginning of this book that I am one of these people who must struggle on a regular basis to keep my belly in shape. So this book is both a professional discussion of how I work with clients who want to deal with their midsection condition, and also a personal exploration of how I have dealt with my own question of belly consciousness and fitness.

There is perhaps nothing more important to a man than his relationship with his belly region because this is the physical and emotional center of a person's being. Our minds and hearts certainly orchestrate our feelings and ideas, but the primal origins of our personal power and emotional expression are located deep down in our very guts, as we all know from experience. So it makes practical sense to devote a book to this theme.

But I want to say right at the start that there

is no ideal image of a physical belly that I hold in mind as I write this book. Each of us has a unique body structure, and also a unique personality, and it is the combination of these two attributes that determines our own optimum belly condition.

There is no turning back the clock when it comes to the condition of our belly region. Many men compare their present condition with how they were when they were younger, and then try to regain that youthful shape. But life doesn't work that way. We can move forward into a new relationship with our bellies, but we cannot return to a previous state; this is a reality we must deal with in a positive way, or we will never achieve a more satisfying relationship with our belly.

Each of us ultimately must choose for himself the ongoing size and shape of his belly. Some men are able quite naturally to carry a big belly around as their preferred presence in the world, and I am not making any judgments whatsoever about your personal belly condition or preference. The question is: Did you choose your present belly size and condition, or did it somehow just sneak up on you when you weren't looking?

What I want to do is this—to offer you a practical way to explore your relationship with your belly, physically, emotionally, and on deeper spiritual levels as well. And once you have come to an intimate understanding of how your belly influences your life, I want to offer you practical tools for improving your belly condition, if you choose to act in this direction.

Many times in this discussion, I am going to ask you to consider questions about your relationship with your belly that might seem silly, even embarrassing, or that might prove challenging. But this challenge will be well worthwhile. I want to guide you through the same set of experiences and reflections that we would go through if you came to me as a client wanting some help in dealing with your relationship with your belly. And, by the end of the book, you should find yourself quite deeply grounded in this relationship.

Our bellies are not, of course, static conditions. They are constantly in change, reflecting how we are feeling deep-down emotionally, as well as what we are doing physically in our everyday routines. There are many ways to influence the shapes and conditions of our bellies, and my aim in this book is to teach you these various techniques for helping your belly to evolve in directions you find worthwhile.

In my work as a therapist over the years, I have found that many clients are able to grow and heal emotionally through focusing on their physical belly conditions and working to develop more power and grace in the abdominal regions of their bodies. And, in the opposite direction, most clients find that their physical belly shapes improve as they work through emotional inhibitions.

Introduction

What we are going to do in this program is to approach both ends of the growth spectrum as a unified pair, regularly exploring your emotional activities in your belly while also learning movement and dietary approaches to abdominal fitness. We will be going on several memory expeditions into your childhood and young adulthood, to see what you remember about your belly condition earlier in your life. We will be exploring your unconscious attitudes about your belly and your self-image. And we will also be considering your eating habits, and how these interact with emotional and movement habits to determine your belly shape.

Although dietary and exercise factors do play a part in any belly-fitness program, I personally consider these aspects secondary to the deeper question of how you see yourself in your own mind. If you are rejecting your belly, for instance, and sending hate vibes down there all the time, such mental habits are going to negate any exercise or dietary efforts you might make to flatten your belly.

Basically, my approach to therapy, and to belly fitness as well, is this—first of all we must come to accept and love ourselves just as we are. Then and only then are we in position to encourage an evolution of our whole being in directions that we choose. We simply can't hate our bellies and help them at the same time. We have to reestablish a healthy, acceptant relationship with this part of our bodies if we are going to bring about positive change in this region.

Although I have written this book with a scope that does not pretend to understand women and their bellies as well as I understand my own gender's bellytalk, I do hope that women readers will find this book of interest, both in understanding their men friends better and in seeing the similarities and the differences between a woman's relationship with her belly and a man's relationship with his.

Perhaps the biggest difference between a man and a woman, at belly level, is that a man simply doesn't have a belly that can become full with pregnant portent. Women have quite different muscular configurations in the belly region to accommodate a growing being living within their bellies. The birth process itself also requires certain powerful muscles, which women have and men don't.

In his famous book *Ulysses*, James Joyce created a memorable male character named Bloom, who just happened to carry around quite a good-sized belly. Bloom's belly played a very important role, and as the man came to a deeper and deeper relationship with his big belly, he arrived at the point where he realized that it was in fact an unconscious expression of his desire to have a baby.

Since Bloom was a man and not a woman, his urge to be pregnant was not possible in reality. But he could nonetheless go around with a big belly, which gave him the feeling of being pregnant, and that was better than nothing.

Many men do in fact go around sporting big bellies as if they were a sign of potency. A big belly does often give the impression that its owner is pregnant with some special feeling or potential. To be pregnant with an idea is a very common feeling in men as in women.

I would venture to say that most men with big bellies do gain some positive feeling from having their bellies. They feel physically big, for a starter, and bigness in itself can give a sense of power and well-being. They also feel full instead of empty. For reasons we will explore in depth later on, this question of fullness lies at the heart of a tendency toward a big belly.

Many men with protruding midriffs often insist that they identify with their bellies, that they wouldn't know who they would be without them. This is one of the main reasons why it is sometimes so difficult for a man to get rid of his belly—deep down there is resistance to the very idea.

$$\odot$$

As a beginning contemplation, let me throw out to you the following point to ponder for a few moments, as you put this book aside and focus directly on that belly of yours, regardless of its size right now. Would you be the same man if you

lost your belly? And if, through losing your belly, you became a new person, somewhat as a surprise to you and those around you, are you ready for this transformation? Put your hands on your belly for a few breaths, and see what feelings and insights come to you.

1
Muscletalk

If you go off to the beach on a warm summer's day and walk around casually observing exposed midriffs, you will see quite dramatically that there are as many different belly types as there are people with bellies. Each of us has our own unique posture, our own unique way of holding our belly in, or letting it hang out.

When we speak of the condition of your belly, we are in fact talking about several factors that interact intimately to create the final impression you make on other people when they look at you and your belly.

First of all, your belly appearance depends on how much fat you have allowed to accumulate around your midriff. Whereas women often put on fat in their upper thighs and derrieres, men tend to deposit their extra calories right around the belt line so that there is a noticeable difference in the size of that inner-tube insulation that we call the midriff bulge.

But beyond the simple question of caloric deposits, the size of a man's belly is also determined by the actual size of his stomach and intestines. From chronic overeating and drinking, the intestines become elongated and puffy, and bulge out in front as a result of not having enough room within the abdominal cavity. It is this condition that most directly affects one's health, since a clogged, sluggish digestive tract can lead to all sorts of serious, long-term health problems.

There is a third factor that also determines a man's relative belly size, and this is the strength and tone of the different layers of muscles that hold the intestines in place. In this chapter I want to take time to allow you to explore your relationship with these important muscles so that you can evaluate their present condition, reflect on past experiences that affected their strength or weakness, and see if you want to start to get these muscles in better shape.

Let's go back a moment to your walk along the summer beach in your bathing suit. I'd like you to take a look around the beach until you find some young children playing in the sand. If you pause a moment you will notice that the younger the child, the bigger a belly this child will tend to have. Babies have big bellies when they are upright because they have not yet developed their belly muscles adequately. In fact, until they learn to walk they really only exercise these muscles when they laugh, cry, or breathe.

It's important to reflect on the fact that you were just like these little toddlers, with a big belly sticking out, when you first learned to stand upright and walk about. Babies also very often have a special layer of fat around their bellies, very similar to what men develop again later on.

But most babies start to lose their baby fat, and also begin to develop stronger abdominal muscles, as they start running around and being more active. By the age of three or four most children have solid belly muscles and have lost their early layers of fat. In the process of turning from little angels into little monsters, two- and three-year-olds have transformed themselves from weak dependence into the first stages of a strong, independent maturity.

Many of us, however, carry with us a predisposition to regress to these early baby days, especially if our mothers indulged us overmuch in this stage. And if we fall in love in adulthood with a woman who loves to baby us, it is only natural for us to slip into some of the old patterns of baby times.

You can imagine how carefully I have had to progress with some big-bellied male clients, in order to help them see into the baby aspects of their belly conditions. Most men are seriously offended if someone suggests that they are still on certain levels big babies. This is an ultimate insult to an insecure male ego.

⊙

To what extent are your stomach muscles strong and successful in holding your intestines in place? And, conversely, to what extent have you slipped back into a weak belly state that reflects your tendency to indulge in early childhood feelings? Take a few moments now to reflect on this question.

⊙

There is a particularly pleasurable feeling of weakness in the belly muscles that is associated with infantile feelings, and I suspect that every man feels this weakness now and then. It is, in fact, natural and to be desired, to occasionally indulge in the relaxed, dependent feelings you knew as a baby. Many men have serious troubles in relationships specifically because they cannot occasionally melt into infantile bliss states.

So please don't think that I am judging negatively the relaxed muscular states that you knew as a baby and that you can occasionally indulge in as a grown man. My concern applies only when this muscular condition is chronic, when there is simply not enough strength in the belly muscles to hold the intestines firmly in place while you are moving about.

Optimally, during each day there are times for relaxation and times for tension of the abdominal muscles. For instance, you simply won't be able to drop off into sleep if you have tight stomach muscles. Many men are in such a state of tension that their stomach muscles are chronically tight as a habit, and their ability to relax is undermined as a result. To be able to sleep like a baby is one of the highest attainments in adult life.

At the same time, it is important to be able to have a hard stomach and abdominal stance when you are out facing the dangers and challenges of the world. For many men, a bulging belly with weak abdominal muscles is an external reflection of an inner weakness, which goes right back to difficulties in the first few years of life. I am not going to burden this discussion with psychological theories to this effect. But I do want to stimulate some intuitive reflections within you regarding your past success in learning how to be strong in your belly. We will take some time later on to guide you back into some memories of those early days.

For now, though, I want to turn your attention more to the present moment, to the interaction between your conscious mind and those abdominal muscles we have just been talking about. This relationship between your conscious awareness and your belly muscles will be a primary force in any belly transformations you bring about, because it is only through developing a new mental habit regarding belly-muscle fitness that genuine long-term changes can come into being.

You can make temporary progress in flattening your belly and losing some weight by pushing yourself to go to the gym and forcing yourself to exercise and diet. Many men are pressured by wives and bosses and negative inner feelings into programs to reduce the external manifestation of their belly problems. But all too often, in the long run, these torturous exercise routines and crash diets fail to produce a lasting inner transformation.

Such failure usually comes about when a man tries to change his physical appearance without changing his mental and emotional habits, which generated the physical condition in the first place. And the successful path to a flat and powerful belly is just what we are exploring right now—the combination of conscious inner evolution with enjoyable dietary and movement routines.

Let's take a look at your own relationship with your belly muscles right at this moment. As you continue reading these words, see if you can become aware of the belly muscles that are holding your abdomen in place. Don't make any effort to artificially contract the muscles if you find them weak. Just notice, with each breath, what actual sensations you pick up about the position of your belly and the movements happening as you breathe.

You will notice first of all that there is an intimate relationship between your belly muscles and your breathing. With every inhale, as air comes into your lungs and pushes down on your abdomen, there is an outward movement of your belly. As you exhale and the air rushes out of your lungs, the abdomen has more room and moves back inward somewhat.

If you completely relax your stomach muscles, the inhale is created by the contraction of your diaphragm muscle as it pulls the lungs down, and the exhale is created as the diaphragm muscle relaxes upward and gravity helps to collapse the chest region. Thus, with the abdominal muscles completely relaxed, breathing continues. This is how you breathe in deep sleep, for instance, and it is also the kind of breathing you want to encourage when you need to relax and reduce the stress in your body.

When you must get up and move about, however, you naturally shift into a different way of breathing, one that brings into play your abdominal muscles. You inhale in the same way, but when it is time for your next exhale, you contract your abdominal muscles to help push the air out of your lungs quickly and completely.

Many people with weak belly regions have developed the habit of keeping their abdominal muscles relaxed, rather than contracting them when they exhale. If you have this habit, you will probably want to begin to reverse it, step by step. Let's look directly at your own muscular habits through the following basic belly meditation.

⊙

THE ABDOMINAL EXHALE MEDITATION

With every exhale, consciously contract your belly muscles, to help push the air out of your lungs. After you have exhaled completely, hold your muscles tight a moment to feel this contraction intimately, and then relax the muscles to allow your next inhale to come rushing in. Do this belly breath meditation five or six times as you look away from the book, and begin to expand your conscious awareness of your belly muscles. (If you stand up and walk around as you do this, you will intensify the experience.)

> **Exhale . . . contract your belly muscles**
> **Inhale . . . relax your belly muscles**
> **Exhale . . . contract**
> **Inhale . . . relax**

and continue breathing this way for a few more breaths on your own.

* * *

After doing this breathing—belly muscle exercise, just breathe normally and notice how your belly muscles feel, to open yourself to a new feeling of relationship between your mind and your belly. Do this now, and see what comes to you.

⊙

Although this subtle exercise might seem unimportant at first, you have actually just learned one of the most vital belly routines of all. Too often people think that the only exercises that help flatten the belly are the strenuous ones. But in fact what is most important for a genuine belly transformation is to develop habits for doing more subtle exercises many times during each day.

This particular exercise, which is formally called the *abdominal exhale meditation*, is especially important because you can do it anywhere, anytime, in any state of mind. You can do it in the middle of a business meeting and it will bring you into a calmer, and yet more powerful, state of mind. You can do it while waiting for lunch, or while driving down the freeway. You can equally do it while reading the newspaper or holding your lover. You are breathing all the time, and every time you exhale, you can consciously make contact with your abdominal muscles and give them the gentle order to contract until you are empty of air. Then you give the beautiful order to relax so that the air can rush into your lungs again.

With most clients, I give this beginning breath meditation in the first session, so that we have a concrete and powerful routine available that can be instantly learned and effortlessly integrated into everyday life. It usually does little good to try to begin the belly-transformation process with complicated exercises and meditations. Like all genuine progressions, working to bring about changes in your weight and posture, in your sense of personal power and confidence, requires finding a simple beginning point where you can dig in and gain a successful foothold from which to make further steps.

You now have such a beginning point.

My suggestion is that you do this abdominal exhale meditation for six breaths once an hour for the next ten days, and see if it becomes a habit. If it does, you've just transformed your belly, congratulations. But notice that everything is up to you with this, up to your ability to remember to do the six-breath meditation on a regular basis.

⊙

Try it again for six breaths right now, and see what new experiences come to you and your belly.

2

A Conversation with Your Belly

That noble belly of yours has been working hard for you ever since your very first days on planet earth, digesting whatever you send down its way and dealing appropriately with the burnable stuff and unwanted stuff. The intestinal tract is quite a remarkable mechanism, having been here for as long as living organisms have been populating the world.

But your particular belly is more than just a food-processing plant, it is also a region of your body where emotions are felt, where strength and weakness have their roots in your personality. And it is this combination of emotions and physiological functions that makes the belly such a dynamic entity.

A therapist named Fritz Perls, who began a form of therapy called Gestalt, developed a very effective way for helping people get in touch with their bellies. I want to share with you his techniques, so that you can experience a quite dramatic new relationship with that region of your being.

What I am going to suggest is this: that you carry on various conversations with your belly, in make believe of course, but also quite realistically as you let parts of your body speak that usually are given no voice. At first you might consider such conversations foolish or even impossible, but I think you will quickly catch on to the magic of this process, and enjoy it.

⊙

For instance, why don't you begin with a conversation about the food you eat? First of all, tell your stomach and digestive tract why you ate the food you ate so far today. Explain the nutritive value of the food you ate, the pleasure it gave you, and so on, until you have fully explained to your belly your reasons for eating what you did. (It usually works best to close your eyes while you give this silent explanation. Imagine that your belly is an actual person whom you are talking to.) Try it now.

* * *

And now it is time for you to let your belly talk back to you, with its response and its attitudes toward your eating habits. Perhaps your stomach loves the food you send down for it to deal with, but perhaps it sometimes gets angry with you for what you eat and the amount you eat. Let your belly express its emotions as well as its opinions about how you treat it.

Now you get to talk back to your belly and explain why you treat it the way you do, and also to respond to any new insights you've gained through listening to its side of the story.

Finally, let your belly tell you what sort of treatment it would ideally prefer from you. What sorts of food would be best for it to handle, for instance, and what quantities?

Now you can put your stomach aside for the moment, and talk for a while with all the fat that might have accumulated around your midriff. Express your feelings of love, of anger, of hatred even toward the fat you carry. Really let your fat know how you feel about it, as you close your eyes and speak out loud or to yourself, whichever you prefer.

Now switch positions, and let your fat speak back to you with whatever reactions it might have to what you said to it. See how your fat feels about

your desire to destroy its very existence, and your prejudices against its presence.

⊙

I recommend that you carry on these conversations with your stomach and intestines and fat a number of times, with a few days between conversations. You will notice that every time you pause to talk to your belly or your fat, new feelings and attitudes will have evolved. In fact, you will need to continue talking with your belly and your fat for the rest of your life if you want to maintain a healthy relationship with them.

Let me share with you a sample conversation that I have monitored between a client and his belly and fat, so you can get more of a feeling for what I am suggesting you explore with your own belly and fat.

Tom: *I don't like you, Belly. You stick out there and embarrass me all the time. Girls look at me and make ugly faces, as if I'm totally ugly, just because you're down there with your big ugly bulge, ruining everything for me. And I hate how weak you are too. Why don't you get yourself in shape and stop ruining my life?*

Tom's Belly: *Listen to you talk, you with your big mouth that eats everything it can get its hands on, you with the weak mind that makes me feel weak too! It's not my fault that you've stuffed me so full of meat and cheese and candy and alcohol and all the rest that I can't burn everything you send down here. It's all your fault!*

Tom: *You don't have to shout so loud. There you go again, causing trouble for me. What if people hear what you're saying? Then they're going to have a still worse opinion of me.*

Tom's Belly: *I think you have a worse opinion of yourself than anyone else has of you.*

Tom: *That's not true. Well, I don't think it's true.*

Tom's Belly: *And why are we fighting all the time like this? You never give me any help so I can get in better shape, you know. All you do is blame me for everything, and expect me to somehow change my looks. But we've got to do it together, you and me. You've at least got to pay me enough attention so that you notice when I'm trying to communicate with you.*

Tom: *I listen to you. You're always telling me you're hungry, you're hungry. And so I feed you, and look what you do to me: You get big, you put on all that fat, and then nobody likes me.*

Tom's Belly: *Oh poor you, poor you. What about me? I'm down here ready to get really sick, you know. My linings are clogged so bad with all that junk you eat that I can hardly get anything through the old pipelines. And you're drinking so much beer that I'm always just in terrible shape down here. What about cutting down a little?*

Tom: *Maybe I don't have the discipline to cut*

down on things like you want me to. It's not easy up here dealing with the outside world, you know. All you have to do down there is sit around and digest. You don't have to deal with the stress of the outside world.

Tom's Belly: *Well, that's a joke too. Every time you get upset, you completely ruin my digestive work down here. That's something else I've been wanting to tell you. You've got to get some kind of control over your moods, and stop being upset so much of the time; it's half the reason I can't digest the food properly.*

Tom: *Just tell me how I'm supposed to change my life, since you seem to be full of advice.*

Tom's Belly: *Maybe you and I could be better friends, for a starter. You don't do either of us any good when you're always blaming me for everything. We could work together as a team and help each other out, be each other's best friend. After all, we're in this together, whether we like it or not.*

Tom (after a pause): *Hmm. I guess we are. But you know I tried to make things better for us. I fasted last month for two days and—*

Tom's Belly: *—and then you ate two cartons of ice cream on the third afternoon and about killed both of us, remember?*

Tom: *Okay, so I'm not perfect. But what can I do that will help?*

Tom's Belly: *I know it's no use suggesting that you go to the gym three times a week and totally* change your diet, although those two things would be what I would recommend. But at least you could make some small step, and stick to it, and start a long-term movement in the right direction.

Tom: *Okay, I'll do my best. But where should I start?*

Tom's Belly: *Start with that abdominal exhale meditation you just learned. Do you remember it?*

Tom: *Vaguely.*

Tom's Belly: *I noticed that you didn't get up and walk around while you did the exercise.*

Tom: *The book said I didn't have to if I didn't want to.*

Tom's Belly: *That's your trouble right there, you just don't want to make an effort at all to help us.*

Tom: *So nobody's perfect.*

Tom's Belly: *I'm getting really irritated with that excuse from you all the time.*

Tom: *I feel silly just walking around contracting my belly muscles.*

Tom's Belly: *Maybe someone would see you with your belly held in for once, and you'd make a good impression.*

Tom: *Hmm, I didn't think of that. And anyway, even when I do contract my belly muscles, there's still all that fat down there.*

Tom's Belly: *You've got to make the first step. You can't expect miracles.*

Tom: *Well, it's going to take a miracle to get rid of you and all that fat. I hate that fat!*

Tom's Belly: *Have you ever considered the fact that your fat doesn't like you all that much either?*

Tom: *Why wouldn't my fat like me?*

Tom's Belly: *Maybe you should have a little talk with your fat and find out for yourself.*

Tom: *Hmm, not a bad idea. Hey, Fat, can you hear me, you ugly hunk of whale blubber?*

Tom's Fat: *Watch what you call me or I'll put on two more pounds.*

Tom: *Oh, well, pardon me. But I was just wanting to open up communication with you, because I want you to go away.*

Tom's Fat: *That's not a very friendly attitude toward your very own fat.*

Tom: *Well, let me rephrase my feelings . . .*

3
Remembering Slimmer Days

There are, of course, three dimensions to the story of you and your belly. First of all, there is the present moment, the one you are experiencing right now, while you are reading this book and seeing what transformations come about day by day. Second, there is that vast, uncharted region of your future, in which your belly will get bigger and more out of shape, remain basically the same as it is now, or become smaller and stronger, more in harmony with the rest of your being.

And third, there is that equally vast universe of your personal past, during which your belly went from infant to young child to teenager to young adult to wherever you may be now. Although my

27

primary aim in therapy, and in this book as well, is to help people come more fully into the present moment, where in fact everything is continually being transformed from future through present into past, I am also deeply aware that reflections on one's past can provide vital understanding of the mystery of the present moment.

You will probably be somewhat amazed that even though you have been living with your belly quite intimately for many years, you will at first have some difficulties tapping into memories related to your belly. People with midriffs that they are not happy with tend to block out of memory anything having to do with the development of their present bellies. So it can take a little time before you gain access to the memories I will be aiming you toward.

I would like to say a word at this point about this question of time itself. Most people these days feel somehow constantly time pressured, as if there is simply not enough time to get everything done that they want to get done. Therefore, I know that most readers of this book will be reading rapidly, wanting to gather information quickly, to get done with the book as rapidly as possible. There is, of course, no actual time pressure being applied to you concerning you and your stomach (unless your girlfriend or boss has given you an ultimatum to lose it by Friday or else!). But we are so programmed, from the cradle up, to automatically impose this time pressure on ourselves that our reading habits are locked into this chronic rushing syndrome.

My response to this habitual time pressure is, it's okay if you choose to read through this book quickly, skipping over the meditations and exercises. I have purposely made the text fairly short, so that you can knock the book off in an evening if you so desire.

But at some point you probably will want to take up the book again, perhaps devoting an evening to each chapter, to see how deeply you can delve into the experiences I am suggesting. I hope my ideas and insights can give you a little help in themselves. But it is only through taking time to go into your own inner relationship with your belly that genuine growth can occur. And certainly with the movement exercises I am going to suggest, you will simply have to discard your notion that something can happen overnight if you want to make realistic progress with your physical condition in the midriff.

The beautiful thing about personal evolution is this: You have the rest of your life to do it, and no one is standing around testing your evolutionary speed. Once you realize this, you can take a good, deep breath and relax into the enjoyment of organically sound progression.

If it is going to take time to transform your relationship with your belly, then the logical next step is to make sure that you enjoy every moment of this progression you are involved in. Since in reality you can have no certainty about where you are ultimately heading, it makes excellent sense to focus on enjoying every step along the way. I hope that you share my interest in the present moment enough to see if you can in fact find space and time opening up for you as you do these meditations and movement routines.

⊙

For instance, let's return our focus to your past. Think of all the moments that have gone by since you were born. How many of those moments did you relax into and enjoy? Pause a few breaths if you want to, if you have time to, close the book, close your eyes if you want to, and see how many memories come to you, of times when you were in a relaxed state, when your belly felt good, and when you were in harmony with whatever was going on around you.

⊙

That was quite a gigantic memory suggestion, intended simply to open your mind to the free flow of impressions from your past. You can now sharpen your focus by looking back into your past with the following suggestion:

⊙

Remember the shape and general feeling in your belly region the year you graduated from high school. Close your eyes if you want to, breathe in a relaxed way, and let the memories come of themselves.

Were you strong in the belly when you were a teenager, or were you weak?

Did you like the feeling in your belly during this period of your life? See if you can remember the emotions that were predominant when you were a teenager.

⊙

There is, as I have mentioned before, an intimate relationship between your belly condition and your emotional condition at any given point in your life. To look back into various periods of your life and remember your dominant feelings, and your belly condition at the same time, is a good opportunity for insight into your present belly situation.

⊙

See if you can remember the years after school was over, when you went out into the world in one way or another. What happened to the feelings in your belly region again, and how did the appearance of your belly change?

Now I would like to suggest that you remember back to your childhood and look to see what your father's belly was like when you were little. Was your father in good physical condition, or was he somewhat weak in the belly? Close your eyes and see what memories of your father's belly come.

Now see if you can remember what your mother's attitude was toward your father's belly, and men's bellies in general. Did she consider a big belly a sign of weakness or of positive qualities? Just open yourself to whatever memories come of your mother, and see if they shed light on this belly question.

⊙

Let me give you one final memory suggestion, to take you in whatever directions it might stimulate. I want to give you time to put this book aside, close your eyes if it helps, and go back in your past looking for any experiences that come to mind in which you were aware of the feelings in your belly region. You have literally millions of such memories, I am sure. And I recommend that you do this basic belly-memory meditation a couple of times a day, for quite some time to come, to fully explore your past experiences. Such exploration should be fun and surprising, as you suddenly find yourself remembering feelings in your belly region that you had long ago forgotten. Let yourself remember both the beautiful, positive feelings of power and blissful relaxation in the belly and also the times of fear and weakness there.

⊙

Now it is a good idea to round off this memory expedition by coming back fully into the present moment, to see how your belly region is feeling right now. Is there tension in the belly muscles, or relaxation? Do you feel any particular emotions in your belly? Close your eyes for a few moments, and tune in to exactly what is happening in your belly region.

⊙

During the next days and weeks, see if you can remember to pause a few moments now and then, to do this basic memory expedition on your own. There will always be new memories waiting to pop up to the surface of your mind now that you have begun the process of opening yourself to reflections about your belly. Such reflections can be extremely entertaining as well as insightful, as you remember all the bellies you have known in the past and tune in to your own belly experiences as well.

4

Self-Image Alterations

There are two types of men who have very difficult times transforming their belly images. The first consists of the men who refuse to admit that they have big bellies. They negative-hallucinate their bellies into nonexistence and hold on to a self-image of being flat-stomached and strong in the belly. This image is usually carried over from earlier days, when in fact they were in good shape belly-wise. And as long as this false self-image persists, there is no real hope of any changes happening around their midriffs.

The second type of man who has great difficulty in altering the shape and strength of his belly is the one who is afraid to change his self-image, because any projected change evokes an identity crisis. As long as solid resistance to change in self-image exists, the belly will remain unchanged, regardless of superficial efforts to do away with it.

Actually, most men with extended midriffs carry a little of both these types within them. We tend to hold on to our old self-image which was more flattering than our present one. And we cherish our existing sense of who we are rather than face the uncertainty of evolving into a new being. It is essential that we take a look at our habits of resisting change, so that we can see where we hold ourselves back and how we might break free of our resistances so we can move forward in life.

⊙

First of all, let me give you some suggestions that will help you to see clearly your present self-image, with regard to your belly. See what happens if, after reading this paragraph, you put this book aside, close your eyes, and visualize yourself standing about 15 feet away from you. See if you can imagine your body clearly and notice what your image of your belly is.

⊙

Probably you found that you have more than one visual impression of yourself. Most men will first of all see themselves in very fit condition, an ideal self-image. Then they will suddenly see their very worst fears of how they might appear to other people, with a big, weak, bulging belly that looks just terrible. Then they will visualize a number of quick variations on these two themes, until they begin to create a reasonably realistic image of themselves in their minds. Is this somewhat representative of what you just experienced?

⊙

It may be fruitful for you to do this same visualization exercise again right now, to see one step deeper into how your mind plays with the notion of your physical image. Give yourself time, so that your mind can enjoy the visualization process.

⊙

The basic psychological reality seems to be this: Your external physical shape, the posture and fitness of your body, is a reflection of a deep-seated image that you have developed from the time you were born up to the present moment. Unless this mental image actually evolves into a new image of your physical condition, it is almost impossible to bring about the physical changes you are aiming toward. This is why so many men fail in their honest, devoted efforts to get rid of their bellies.

If you deep down see yourself as a weak person, for instance, it will be almost impossible for you to develop a genuinely strong physical presence. You might overwork yourself at the gym to develop giant muscles, you might learn great karate chops with which to impress people around you. But hiding underneath this facade of physical strength will always be your self-image as a weak person.

Unfortunate as the case may be, we are quite capable of fooling both the people around us and even ourselves when we manipulate our external images to pretend to be something that is the opposite of who we are deep down. When I first see a new client who has bulging muscles and a stomach that you could run a truck into without hurting him, I know that we have a tremendous amount of work ahead of us before we can arrive at the level of therapy that helps a weak man become genuinely strong in the belly. With a man who openly shows that he has a weak belly, I can start right away exploring ways in which he can honestly begin to get centered in his strength again. But with a man who refuses to admit to an inner weakness in the belly, it is almost impossible to make any forward steps until the armor has been broken down.

However, if you are reading this book, you probably already honestly admit to yourself that you need to come to better terms with your belly—

so you are one step ahead of the he-man who is fooling even himself regarding his deeper belly feelings. In fact, most overdeveloped muscle men are seriously out of touch with the feelings in their bellies. They have made the belly region so hard and unfeeling that there is a complete lack of connection between belly and emotions.

⊙

Take a break for a few moments right now, and see how this discussion has been affecting the muscles and feelings in your belly.

⊙

What I want to talk about specifically in this chapter is the process through which you can consciously evolve from your present self-image into the self-image you desire. And the first step in this process is to consider the self-image you are hoping to evolve into. You will want to see if this self-image is realistic, if you can in fact make logical steps and attain your goal.

Primarily, you will want to make sure that you are actually creating a new self-image for your future, and not simply projecting your old, youthful self-image onto your future goal. I would venture to say that the vast majority of men who fail in their attempts to transform their belly images fail because they are trying to become what they once were, rather than evolving to become people they have never been before. To become someone new is scary. To try to return to an earlier stage of development appears safe, because it is a known state. But in reality no matter how much we would like to turn back the biological clock, we have no choice but to move forward.

⊙

So let's consider how you would like to look six months from now. After reading this paragraph, let your eyes close if they want to, as you put aside the book for a few moments, tune in to your breathing and your belly, and begin to conjure up an image of yourself as you hope you will look after six months of working with this program. Imagine yourself standing naked in front of you. Notice how your belly looks and how you are feeling in your body.

⊙

How many pounds lighter were you in your imagination than you are now? In six months you can lose a lot of pounds, this is true. But how fast can your self-image lose pounds? I'm sure you know that most men who go on crash diets and lose 20 pounds in as many days almost invariably regain those pounds in the following weeks. As I have mentioned, this is mostly because their bodies lost weight, but their self-image didn't. And the self-image is the actual determining factor in any long-term physical change.

So I prefer the following procedure for losing weight.

⊙

Set about to lose 6 pounds in the next six weeks. And as you lose each pound, meditate on its loss. See if you are willing to become a pound lighter. See if you can let go of this part of yourself. And do this consciously, so that you directly stimulate an alteration in your self-image.

⊙

A self-image is basically a concept in your mind, which has sunk mostly into the unconscious over the years. To alter it, you will need to regularly, every day if at all possible, meditate on that 1 pound that you want to lose in your self-image. If you do this faithfully, you have the best chance of actually losing that pound for good. Then you can move on to the next pound the following week.

I will give some particular dietary suggestions in a later chapter, and some important movement suggestions as well. But let me say that in an extreme instance you can actually meditate away pounds, without doing anything drastic otherwise to your life-style. The mental act is most important. The eating and moving factors come of themselves if the mental evolution is activated first.

Almost all of you will encounter, when you seriously reflect on your desire to alter your self-image, a part of you that fears any change at all. My suggestion for when you encounter this resistant part is this: Become friends with it. Gain a deeper understanding of your fears concerning change. And also be respectful of this hesitant dimension of your personality. There is a good reason why human beings are basically conservative beings. Too much change too fast is a danger to anyone's survival. And too radical a shift in one's self-image can be suicidal. You must remain centered in your existing personality and advance through life step by step, rather than try to grow in one sudden leap into the unknown.

I must admit that ten years ago I would not have written that last paragraph. I used to believe strongly in the ability of human beings to make giant leaps in their evolution. I was a young psychologist during the wild sixties, when we believed people could totally transform themselves in a matter of weeks. But the reality of the human condition proved to be less flexible than we hoped. Human beings can in fact accelerate their evolution, but everything takes place within the structure of time. Evolution is a step-by-step affair. Certainly we advance in growth spurts followed by periods of relative relaxation. But the pace of growth must be organic, and the leaps must be no further than your psychic feet can manage.

So I recommend a pound or two a week, or whatever reasonable goal you choose to give yourself, if you want to lose some pounds from your midriff. And I also suggest that you be easy with yourself if you find this pace too rapid.

What you really want to do is explore the flexibility of your self-image, instead of placing rigid expectations on it. If you don't lose a single pound in six weeks, that is perfectly okay. That means that your self-image was not ready for the alteration, or that in fact it is best for you to stay at your present weight and love yourself just as you are. Whatever you do, don't try to violate the integrity of your self-image, unless you want some very confusing days ahead. If you love yourself, you will accept both your potential for change and your need to remain the same as you are. It is the dynamic of these two opposites that creates the beautiful challenge of growing, throughout your life.

Along with losing pounds, the transformation of your self-image should ideally include strengthening the muscles in your belly region. In fact, these two processes should almost always be intimately linked. Lots of proper movement, together with conscious meditations on the evolution of your self-image, plus a good diet—these are the three foundation posts of a belly-transformation experience.

And if you don't develop a mental image of yourself as stronger than you are at present, you are going to have little luck in generating true strength in your belly region. So you will want to regularly reflect on the feelings of strength and weakness in your belly while you are doing some of the muscle-building exercises I will be outlining later on. It is essential that you get to know your feelings of weakness in the belly, without rejecting these parts of your overall personality.

We all have weak sides to our inner makeup. We all know anxiety and apprehension, and we universally share the tendency to regress to infantile feelings of helplessness and passivity. What I am suggesting is that you consciously allow these feelings to be a part of your evolving self-image. Then you can make realistic progress with your belly transformations.

⊙

Give this a try right now. Close your eyes after reading this paragraph, relax, and let yourself feel total weakness in your belly region for a few breaths. Surrender to all the buried feelings of

hopelessness and despair inside you, and notice how these feelings affect your belly muscles.

⊙

Very often in therapy work, I lead a client back in his life to remember traumatic experiences in which he was overwhelmed by feelings of total despair and hopelessness. Such experiences, instead of being accepted and let go of, are often denied after they happen. The result of such denial is a lingering weakness in the belly, because the old feelings are always trying to be felt adequately so that they can be discharged and eliminated.

We store many of our old traumatic feelings in our abdominal muscles. When a baby cries, it contracts the gut muscles powerfully and repeatedly, until the physical manifestation of an emotional trauma is fully discharged. But when we grow old enough to block our spontaneous discharges of crying, we start to store these unreleased feelings in the muscles of the belly. Wilhelm Reich, that great early pioneer in emotional release therapy, showed clearly that old traumas continue to influence one's feelings in the belly, until the traumas are finally relived and released through actual contractions of the belly muscles.

Thus with every belly contraction that you consciously cause, be it through emotional expression or physical exercise, you are helping to break free of old, buried feelings and to bring your muscles more into the present moment.

But always, until you actually alter your self-image and your belly condition, there will be two voices talking to you: one telling you that you want to change, the other telling you that you like yourself just as you are.

⊙

Try this: Say to yourself several times, "I want to change my belly."

Now say to yourself, "I don't want to change at all, I like myself just as I am."

Go back and forth from one statement to the other several times, and let yourself feel the honest emotions behind each.

⊙

Let me give you a realistic first step to see if you are ready to alter your self-image in directions you choose. Decide that at least once an hour for the next week you are going to do the abdominal exhale meditation, so that you make regular conscious contact with the belly muscles you want to strengthen.

Also, see if you can begin the following routine to burn calories and strengthen your belly muscles.

If you can make this first step of doing a simple and enjoyable movement routine each morning and evening, you are well on your way to expanding this routine to more powerful stages.

⊙

1. **First of all, simply run in place or around the house for however long you want to, without pushing yourself overmuch. This will get your heart beating powerfully and move you into an altered sense of who you are activity-wise.**

2. **Then lie down on the floor on your back, with both your knees bent and your feet flat on the floor. Straighten one leg, and, as you exhale with a belly contraction, raise that leg slowly into the air. Then, as you inhale, lower the leg slowly to the floor, without quite letting it touch. Raise again on the next exhale, being sure that you are consciously contracting your belly muscles so you feel them strongly. Inhale the leg down again, and repeat this as many times as you want to.**

   Then shift to the other leg, raising it on the exhale, lowering on the inhale, as many times as you want to. Make any variations on this exercise that come to you. The purpose is to really wake up your

belly in a pleasurable way, so do the leg
lifts in whatever way that feels good to
you.

3. Then just relax completely, legs out-
stretched on the floor, and put both hands
on your belly region. As you breathe effortlessly, experience the feelings flowing
through your body, and open yourself to
whatever insight might come to you regarding your self-image and your belly.

⊙

With these three basic steps, you have a complete
minibelly-transformation program that you can do
in just a few minutes. The challenge is this: Watch
yourself during the next few days, and see if you
are ready to do such a program to help alter your
self-image and belly condition, or if there is
resistance.

If you do encounter inner resistance, this is
what you should do: Sit for three minutes each
morning and watch yourself *not* doing your belly-
transformation routine. Just accept yourself as you
are, and watch what goes on inside you. This can be
an enlightening experience. You will finally be able
to see firsthand the old inhibitions and habits that
have, all this time, been keeping you from doing
anything positive to help your belly. And in the process of seeing clearly these mental habits, you will

find them changing. I will speak more of this later.

But consider what you have thus far: You have a beginning understanding of how you can act, concretely, to alter both your inner self-image and your physical condition. You also have the freedom to explore your readiness to make a single, simple step toward improving your belly condition, without having to feel pressured by any success-failure syndromes. So I offer you this beginning program to play with, and hope you gain many insights.

Let me repeat the basic ingredients that make up this positive daily action toward improving your belly condition.

$\odot$

1. **Do the abdominal exhale meditation about once an hour, no matter what else you might be doing.**
2. **Take five minutes to do a simple movement program to strengthen your belly region:**

    a. Run in place as long as you want to, or run around your house or block, feeling your belly muscles as you run.

    b. Lie down on your back and do some single-leg lifts in such a way as to awaken your belly muscles. Do variations on this general theme, such as double-leg lifts, until you are ready to stop.

3. Then relax, focus on your breathing and the feeling in your belly region, and do one of the inner belly meditations that you have learned. Perhaps remember past times with your belly, or contemplate your present self-image or your projected future self-image. You can also carry on your ongoing discussion with your belly, or just focus on whatever emotions might be in your belly region and see if you can let these feelings rise up and out in emotional release.

4. Also, as a general belly-awareness meditation, see if you can be conscious of your belly region throughout every moment of every day, so that your whole life becomes integrated into the ongoing drama of you and your belly.

⊙

There they are, four steps you can take daily that will definitely bring about a transformation of your belly. See how you respond to this program. Watch yourself, explore your readiness to act and also your resistance to acting. Be sure to move gently into this important first belly-transformation program, and enjoy whatever insights come to you every new day.

5

Your Warrior Spirit

In this chapter I want to look directly at a dimension of human tradition that is often ignored or judged quite negatively these days. I am speaking of the fact that men in all cultures have had, as one of their primary identities, that of warrior. Whether we like it or not, human beings have been fighting for their survival, and the survival of their families and communities, for as long as history extends into the past.

In the same way that baby kittens and puppies, baby monkeys and jackrabbits wrestle with one another and their parents, young human children include regular mock fighting as a natural aspect of their growing-up experience. Whether this is more a genetic or a learned behavior is a

question the psychologists will argue about for-
ever. The obvious fact remains: Fighting is part of
our nature. We struggle to hold our own in a world
that would otherwise run over us. A man must
stand strong if he is to maintain his sense of re-
spect, and he must be ready to fight to defend his
home ground and family if he is threatened by outside forces.

⊙

**The question of a man and his belly is intimately
connected to the question of a man and his warrior spirit. Consider for a moment your own image of a noble warrior in the classical traditions.
Imagine, for instance, a Japanese samurai warrior standing in front of you with his lethal sword.
Take a look at this magnificent man's belly region. What condition is it in?**

**Now imagine a mighty American Indian warrior
riding bareback across the plains, bow and arrow
in hand. What is the condition of this warrior's
belly, compared with yours?**

**And now see what your imagination comes up
with concerning your own special childhood
hero, who you worshiped and imagined being
when you were outside playing with your friends
in one of your youthful games of war. Close your**

eyes if this helps in your remembering, and get back in touch with your own belly feelings when you were a wild young warrior.

⊙

The key to being a warrior in modern times is in fact no different from what it was in the old days of physical confrontations. A man's power still resides deep down in his belly, whether he be a samurai warrior or an executive warrior. Power is something that requires both an emotional and a physical readiness to fight for what you think is right. And this power includes a muscular strength in the belly, an emotional strength throughout the body, and a more subtle warrior spirit, which carries on the human tradition that has been passed from generation to generation in all enduring communities. With this in mind, I want to turn your attention back to where you learned this warrior tradition in your own community.

⊙

First of all, consider your father. Did he carry this warrior spirit strong within him? Was he an honest man who fought cleanly, who was not afraid to confront dangers, who knew how to

harden himself and to muster all his inner strength when necessary? Pause a few moments, close your eyes if you want to, breathe into your feelings right now, and see what memories come of your father as a warrior.

If your father had a weak belly and a deteriorated warrior spirit, how did this affect the development of your own warrior spirit? To what extent did you inherit your father's particular stance in life? Again, take some time to reflect on this vital question.

⊙

It is true that some men with weak bellies picked up that condition from identifying with fathers who were also weak as warriors. If this is your life story, then you will need to consciously begin to let go of your identification with your father, so that you can move forward into a new self-image that breaks free of your family inheritance.

But sometimes sons of powerful fathers develop weak bellies. Why is this so? Sometimes a young boy is overwhelmed by the power of his father. Sometimes a father frightens his son too much with the warrior spirit, at too early an age. Then the son reacts by identifying instead with his mother, who is softer, more loving, more understanding of a little boy's needs and limitations.

In fact, perhaps a majority of the men I have worked with as clients who had difficulties in mustering their warrior spirits have been men with overly powerful and frightening fathers, fathers who never gave their sons the chance to develop their own budding warrior spirits step by step. A little boy needs to feel his own strength as adequate. When a father is always overwhelming the boy, the boy's belly feelings of power and self-assertion are not able to develop properly.

The son in this case is always pushed into playing the weak, submissive role. Whenever the son fights back against an overly dominating father, the father uses his superior power to overwhelm the son. The result is the son's self-image of fear, impotence, and submission. The only path to success is seen as that of surrender. This boy will usually develop more devious ways of fighting and winning, while keeping his belly muscles lax so as not to provoke his father.

This, of course, is an infinitely complex question of personality development, and each of us has our own special story of how we learned either to stand as a young warrior or to lie down as a victim. What I want to encourage in you through this discussion is direct reflection on your past history in this regard. You know your own story, if you take time to honestly look in this direction.

⊙

So once again, pause from reading this book, and look back to see what new insights might come to you regarding your relationship with your father or father figures. Did your father let you stand up and be strong, or were you punished and frightened into surrendering your warrior spirit?

⊙

Now we can consider that belly of yours right now, as you are reading these words. Are you able these days to rise to the occasion and be a warrior when necessary, or are you somehow out of touch with this human spirit?

Give the following exercise a try if you want to, either now or as soon as you have an opportunity to do so.

⊙

Stand calmly, and focus on your breathing. Walk around the room slowly but with a growing sense of your personal power. Exhale with slow power. Enjoy an increase of physical presence and alertness, and see how your feeling in your belly changes as you walk around in touch with your warrior spirit.

⊙

See if you can do whatever you have to do next today while remaining conscious of your warrior spirit. This can be an immensely wonderful feeling to begin to nurture as a constant quality in your moment-to-moment experience. I have already given you the basic keys to activating your personal power: Exhale slowly and competely with the abdominal muscles, so that you drop down to your root of power, in your abdomen. And stay in touch with that proud, confident warrior spirit that you knew as a child. Give this a try now as you put the book aside and explore your personal power in action.

6

On Men Counting Calories

In this chapter I want to talk with you about ways for altering your diet so as to drop pounds on a somewhat regular basis.

First of all, let me say that I am not an avid fan of counting calories. For a few weeks this can be worthwhile, as you learn directly what foods give you most of your calories. But once you have learned which eating habits are fattening for you, you can put your calorie list away and focus on actually eating less of those particular foods. This involves discipline, and a little discipline is healthy for all of us.

So I do recommend, if you have not done this already, that you count your calorie intake devotedly for a couple of weeks, to get to know intimately what in fact you are eating. You can get a list of food calories almost anywhere these days, at health-food stores, bookstores, from your wife or girlfriend.

Once you have educated yourself in this regard, you can put the calorie list aside and make a general list of the foods you know are not healthy for you. And, step by step, see what happens to your personality and self-image as you develop some discipline in saying "no thanks" to the foods that you know are unhealthy and fattening.

Let me tell you what I have on my bad-food list, and you can compare it at some point with your opinion about your own eating habits.

First of all, there is no doubt that many men have beer bellies because they drink too much beer. I was just talking with a carpenter about this. He eats a mostly healthy diet, exercises immensely compared with the average guy, and yet still sports a beer belly. The reason is simple. After work he and the guys drink a few beers apiece every evening before going home to dinner. And those few beers a day, with quite a few added over weekends, are responsible for the development of a large fat layer on an otherwise powerful body.

Wine is similar in effect. Same with hard alcohol.

If you drink a lot and have a big belly, or even drink less and have less of a belly, you're going to have to cut back on the drinks if you want to lose the belly. Exercise and dieting on other fronts can help, but ultimately that extra 500 to 1,000 calories a day you take in from drinking are going to keep your belly intact unless you cut out the liquor. Some of you can consciously decide to drop the drinking and enjoy the fresh new life that comes when the fog disappears. Others of you might need to seek some semiprofessional help in guiding you out of the rather insidious grip of alcohol, if you are in fact in it. There are sources you can turn to for help if you feel you need it. And the exercises and meditations on your belly in this program should provide a solid groundwork in this regard as well.

Now as far as food goes, let me say this: Anything that is fried is deadly. Whenever you can, choose food that has not been fried at all. I cannot emphasize this too strongly, from a medical point of view. When you fry animal fat especially, the fat is changed into molecules that are extremely hard to digest and that are prime candidates for ending up as fat molecules in your own body rather than being burned and eliminated from your system. Make a list of all the fried foods you regularly eat, and see if you can say no to them more and more as the weeks and months go by.

Second, of course, dairy products are high on the negative list. Cheeses of all kinds should be avoided like the plague—but, at the same time, I must say that to avoid them completely usually ends up as failure in your diet, as you regress to a heavy cheese diet to compensate for time lost.

Just be conscious of every time you put cheese and dairy products of all kinds in your mouth, and say to yourself, "I'm eating something that makes me fat; can I do without this taste rush?"

As a third grouping of fattening foods, there is the sugar-rush conglomeration of desserts to consider. When you order hot apple pie with ice cream for dessert, just remember that it has more calories than a whole healthy meal.

It is one thing for me to say cut out these foods and let yourself feel a little hungry after dinner. It is quite another thing for you to accomplish this. Let me give you a few concrete suggestions that work for me, that should point you in the right direction.

There are many things you can eat that do taste good and satisfying and yet have low calorie contents. To learn what these foods are is like a blessing to someone wanting to drop some pounds and yet not wanting to suffer in the process.

GOOD, SATISFYING LOW-CALORIE MEALS

If you want to lose weight, you are going to need to drop your calorie intake to about 1,200 calories a day. This means you can eat, for instance, the following:

In the morning, a breakfast of yogurt, fruit, and granola can be satisfying, with a cup of herb tea. (Avoid caffeine while dieting or you'll speed yourself up and get too hungry too soon.) If you have a blender or food processor, take some frozen berries and bananas or any other fruit, grind them up, add low-fat yogurt in a bowl, then some granola, and you have a low-calorie breakfast that will satisfy you. If the yogurt is your main dairy intake of the day, it is a healthy intake of just enough animal fat.

For lunch, cook up a good bowl of brown rice, which will taste excellent if you are in fact hungry. The key to enjoying healthy foods is to get hungry before eating them—then you can break free of junk-food habits and return to the natural foods that help normalize your intestinal tract. Along with the brown rice, you can have either a green salad with lots of raw vegetables or a cooked vegetable, such as cauliflower or spinach, both of which have minimal calories.

Now here is where you can indulge and get away with it—go ahead and put some butter on your rice if you like, some good salad dressing on your salad, some Parmesan cheese on your spinach or cauliflower, so that it tastes good. Yogurt also makes an excellent addition to vegetables. In moderate amounts these condiments add maybe a hundred calories to the meal, but they make you feel like you're really indulging, even though the meal only runs up to about 500 calories if you drink lemon water instead of beer or Coke or milk. (Spring water with a good slice of lemon is, along with being calorie free, one of the best drinks in existence.)

With this breakfast and lunch, you have eaten 400, or, at the most, 500 calories per meal, totaling about 900 for the day thus far. This means you can have a snack at three or four, and dinner, if you eat the right foods, and stay below 1,200 calories a day total.

For a snack, I recommend Chinese green tea, which is a powerful red-blood rejuvenator. The tea gives you a healthy boost of energy and becomes a good routine in the afternoon if you have time for it in your day.

Along with the tea, you could have crackers made of rice (Baked Brown Rice Snaps), which have only 7 calories apiece and are available with various flavorings so they serve as a good replacement for junk-food chips. Once again, if you are genuinely hungry, you will find their flavor very good and satisfying.

Add to the crackers (which you can find in health-food stores, imported from Japan) some carrot slices, or other vegetable slices, and you have a balanced and satisfying snack. You can eat seven or eight crackers, by the way, and the total of the snack will still be below 100 calories, whereas a single candy bar will run you well over 200 calories, and a single Coke well over 100 without giving you the satisfaction and the ritual pleasures of a healthy snack.

For dinner, it is wise to eat early and light, so that your stomach isn't loaded with heavy stuff when you head for bed. People with big bellies almost invariably have the habit of eating late and heavy, wolfing down steaks and potatoes at the worst possible hour of the day.

Dinner is time for vegetables or salad, whichever you didn't eat for lunch. You're lucky if you like chopped spinach, because for dinner you can just boil yourself a whole frozen carton, drain it, put it on a warmed plate, add some Parmesan cheese, maybe some gomasio (roasted and salted sesame seeds), a touch of butter, or yogurt, whatever makes it taste like a full meal to you. A whole packet of spinach thusly seasoned will fill you right up if you eat slowly, and it only adds 100 to 150 calories to your count for the day. A good salad adds about the same, unless you get heavy into blue-cheese dressings.

My suggestion if you want something hot to drink after dinner is Bambú, a Swiss noncaffeine drink similar to coffee. It's the only coffee substitute that I can drink with the same pleasure and regularity as coffee. And, once again, I want to clarify that coffee or tea or Coke, anything with caffeine in it, will reduce your ability to fast because the caffeine will make you shaky by burning calories too fast and then give you a craving for junk foods, which will blow your fast instantly.

So there you have my personal approach to dropping down to 1,200 calories a day and enjoying eating every meal. But again, I want to let you in on my own sense of moderation with this diet. You can eat this way through the weekdays, but then on Saturday or Sunday give yourself a big steak or whatever you prefer for lunch or early dinner, with a couple of glasses of wine or beer thrown into the bargain if you want. I have found that I can go for weeks, even months eating very healthy meals during the week if I give myself those weekend splurges to satisfy the part of me that genuinely loves to wolf down a steak now and then.

Balance is all, in the long run.

So find your own way of developing a similar routine for eating as you explore the low-calorie foods you enjoy, and learn how to cook them so that you enjoy them, with a few luxury condiments included to make your taste buds happy. You can also add a piece of chicken during the week for one of your meals, and a piece of fish for another meal if you want more protein in your diet.

⊙

Pause and consider how you feel about eating in this way, eating perhaps 25 percent less, and eating quite different, more healthy, lower calorie foods most of the time.

⊙

A warrior of any sort can go for days without eating anything at all, and with nothing to drink but water, and feel in excellent spirits and very strong and fit. Our bodies can do wonderfully well without constant feeding. We can in fact fast for three days, even seven, even fourteen, without any adverse effects on our bodies. In fact, fasting purifies our systems the natural way.

In most cities these days, there are fasting centers that will teach you how to succeed with a fast, and I strongly recommend that you do such a fast if you want to move quickly into a more powerful, lighter self-image and body shape.

You can also start fasting one day a week, as many traditional societies used to encourage. Take Sunday, for instance, and just don't eat that day. Doing this will reduce your caloric intake by 14 percent or so, while also cleansing your system of toxins you have eaten the previous week.

RUNNING ON EMPTY

The major point of this chapter is that you can shift from running on overstuffed all the time to running on empty, or what will feel at first like empty but will then become a satisfying, full feeling at half the calories. This is a great challenge—to shift your self-image from that of a person who craves food and has to be stuffed to be content to that of a person who likes feeling light, who enjoys being less than full, who can face emptiness and thrive on living a life that is lean, lightweight, controlled, and healthy.

What is wrong with being empty part of the time? Why do we run away from being hungry? And how can we break free of old habits and fears of being hungry, so that we can become in a sense born again, into a new self-image that allows us to feel better and healthier?

Instincts make us associate hunger with the threat of starvation; this is obvious. So it is normal to fear hunger pangs and to hunt for food when we are becoming relatively empty. But the challenge of conscious beings is to understand our instincts, to live within their parameters but also to control our instinctual urges in such a way as to optimize our health and vitality.

This is what I am suggesting in this book—a regular evolution of your self-image so that you are running the show of your life, rather than being pushed around by past conditionings and generalized instinctual urges.

Take the question of the food you eat—it can become a warrior's challenge to face hunger unafraid when you know that you are not in danger of starvation. Be brave, breathe into emptiness when you feel it, relax and eat less at the table, and become a champion who is not addicted to junk food and alcohol. Give up one junk food each new week, for instance, until there are none left in your diet. I challenge you!

7

Flat-Belly Movement Routines

Human beings are perhaps most clearly defined by the ways in which they regularly move about on the planet. In the old days of primitive hunting life, the average man would walk and run perhaps 20 or 30 miles each day. We are in fact magnificent running machines, when we are in shape. And you will look in vain for a big belly on a regular runner.

But these days we move about mostly in cars and buses and trains and airplanes and other variations on effortless themes of transportation. Technology has triumphed over the flat belly and the fit man, creating instead the lethargic commuter, who arrives home at night less fit than when he left home in the morning. What a tragic twist of fate, that we gained the whole world and lost our health.

But I'm sure you know all about this development in your own life.

⊙

Can you remember early days of running running running? Give yourself a few moments you will enjoy, to pause and close your eyes and see what memories come to you of those years when you were a whirlwind of movement. Let the memories come effortlessly, as you simply watch your breathing for a few breaths and turn your attention to your early years on your fast feet.

Now consider how your movement habits started to slow down as you grew older. Look back and remember an average day when you were in high school. What did you do throughout that day that was movement oriented? How much of the day did you sit around? How much of the day were you walking? And how much of the day were you running, dancing, and so on?

And now consider your present movement habits. Go through the list you just used: sitting, walking, running and dancing, and so on.

Also think about your attitude these days toward movement. Do you like to run, for instance? Do you enjoy dancing? Do you like to participate in

sports that get your heart pounding as you run around?

⊙

Obviously, I am encouraging you to begin to increase your movement habits during your regular day. But why is movement so important in regard to your belly condition? First of all, you use your belly muscles when you move. Every time you lift a leg to take a step, you use belly muscles. And when running, you feel the integration of your belly muscles with all the rest of the muscular structure of your body.

Second, as you know for yourself, movement burns calories and helps to burn off the fat that you're carrying around in your midriff. Walking at a quick pace is considered almost as good exercise as jogging. But my experience is this. If you want to tap into your warrior spirit and at the same time lose weight and flatten your belly, you should regularly kick into a higher gear than walking.

Somehow a man is transformed when he breaks into a jogging pace. There is a definite spirit that comes into him that is simply not present otherwise. This is one of the deepest aspects of a human's inherited personality. When you are running, energy comes into the body, and a level of consciousness comes into being that does not exist when you are walking or standing still, sitting or lying down.

But once again, please don't think I am telling you that you have to become a marathon runner, that you have to go out and kill yourself in order to tap into this warrior power and flat-belly transformation.

This is how I went running today. I walked for about two minutes, seeing how I was feeling in my body. In fact, I was feeling heavy, not really wanting to go for a run. There is almost always a certain amount of lethargy and inertia that must be overcome before you tap into your altered nature as a fast-footed warrior.

This push does require a certain amount of discipline. I pushed myself a little into putting on my jogging shoes and getting outside. Just walking outside brought my spirit to a higher level. Then I made the second little push and started a slow lope down the back road. In only ten or fifteen seconds, my heart was pounding harder, adrenaline hit my system, and I felt the transformation occur.

But I didn't force myself to run for an hour without stopping. Instead, I ran for about five minutes, then let myself ease up into a walk, so that I could look around me and tune in to how I was feeling after that running spurt. I could feel my belly tight, my spirit light and energetic. And then, after walking for a couple of minutes, my feet just naturally started running again, and I went back into that heightened state of warrior energy that I love so much.

What I am saying is this: For most men, it is best to eat good food and exercise more, rather than to diet overmuch and stay sluggish in movement habits. I think we can function on just about any diet if we exercise enough. And the curious thing is that when you exercise a lot, you naturally start craving more wholesome foods to eat. Your body is no dummy, given half a chance to regain its organic balance.

So I highly recommend getting outside and running, as much in the country as possible. Get in touch with your childhood spirit of running, and let this transform your present self-image into a mature warrior who still runs. We tend to think that it is somehow childish to be seen running. Especially in the city business clothes many of us have to wear to work, it is almost impossible to break into a run, and if you do so in a city environment, people will look at you as if you are crazy and certainly consider you improper in your behavior. We are extremely lucky to have progressed to where many men do jog regularly these days, of course. Unfortunately, we have turned jogging into a fad instead of letting it exist as a natural thing that men (and women, of course, too) love to do.

Avoid the problems of jogging. Don't do it like a maniac. Give yourself time to have fun. Don't turn it into just another need-achievement ordeal. But be suspicious of the people who say that jogging is dangerous for your knees and so on and so forth. In moderation, with common sense, you can, almost all of you, get out and gently begin to tap back into your wild, free running spirit.

Along with running, I have found that it is very important for a man with a belly to do some specific movement routines that powerfully awaken and strengthen the belly muscles. Let me describe some of the most important belly-specific exercises to you now, so that you can start practicing them on your own if you haven't encountered them before.

While you are trying these movements out for yourself to feel how they awaken your belly region, hold in mind that the trick to a successful movement routine is to find how to move in a way that feels good. Making contact with their various belly muscles does feel good for most people. You only need to learn how to pace yourself so that the pleasure is maximum and the strain minimum. There is a crucial point where you are right on the edge of overdoing the movement and heading into a negative feeling. Be sure to remain sensitive to this point, and back off from it when you reach it. You are not doing these exercises (I hope) to develop monster muscles instantly. Instead, you are doing the movements as a moment-to-moment growing process, in which you and your muscles and your self-image are all exploring the satisfaction of getting in better shape, step by step. The present moment is all. Forget about the future. Enjoy the movement for the pleasure it brings you.

$$\odot$$

LEG LIFTS

I have taught you one basic movement that I hope you have already explored for yourself, leg lifts. Now forget your old associations with this movement. Tap into whatever new experiences come to you as you do it now, in your present level of consciousness. Surprise yourself with the sudden surge of power and pleasure that rushes into your body when you put yourself into stress postures that activate your warrior spirit!

BELLY BENDS

Another posture that will wake up belly muscles in about two seconds is this: Stand with your legs fairly wide apart, toes pointed straight forward. Then slowly bend forward and place your knuckles on the ground below you. Breathe into this powerful posture, and let the energy rush through your belly region. Experiment with different positions of your fists on the floor, to see

how your belly muscles respond. Breathe through the mouth as the power in your body increases to meet the stress of the posture. And then, *before* you reach a point of fatigue, slowly stand up and close your eyes, and breathe into the new feeling you have stimulated in your belly region. Give this a try before we go on, so you can get some experience for yourself: Bend your knees just enough so you can touch the floor, and go down and up several times.

HEAD-TO-FLOOR POSTURE

There are several layers of muscles running in different directions around your abdominal region. To activate some different muscles than you did in the last posture, get down on your knees (on a comfortable rug) and do the following: Slowly lean forward and down until your head touches the ground in front of you, and at the same time raise your arms behind you until they are pointing straight up. Lift your feet off the floor, and look back between your legs as you breathe into this belly-stress posture for as many breaths as feel good to you. Then slowly start to come back to your original kneeling position, feeling intensely how different muscles are activated in different positions. After sitting upright for a couple of breaths of relaxation, move back down into this belly-stress posture again, and

breathe into the feeling. Give this routine a try now, doing it until you are ready to stop.

⊙

The beauty of these movements and stress postures is that every time you do them, you will have a unique experience. You can never get tired of them if you remain in the present moment and breathe into the combination of your emotional and mental state at that moment and the interaction of this state of consciousness with the stress posture you are doing at the time. Once you make contact with this uniqueness of each moment, you will find yourself well on the way to the belly transformations you are desiring.

Hold in mind with each posture and movement that you are consciously waking up the power potential of your belly region, and at the same time are giving yourself the pleasure rush that comes when your warrior spirit is activated deep in your belly.

Try this next routine now if you want to. We're going to tap into some of the martial arts movements that have been used for many generations in the Orient for activating the warrior spirit, but we're going to approach these movements with a balanced lightness that keeps them centered in our own normal state of consciousness.

⊙

WARRIOR ARM MOVEMENTS

Stand with your feet fairly wide apart. Bring your arms straight out in front of you, with the elbows slightly bent. Make a solid fist with each hand. Have your toes pointed straight forward—this is very important, since it determines how the belly muscles will tense in each arm position.

I am now going to describe three different positions to hold your arms in. I want you to inhale and exhale once in each of the positions.

1. **First of all, raise your arms over your head, so that your back arches somewhat and you look up at the ceiling and your clenched fists.**
2. **Now move your arms and fists slowly and consciously downward in front of you, bending your back and knees until your forearms come to rest just above your knees. Inhale and exhale into this position. Hold after the exhale to feel your power in this position.**
3. **Now come upright and bring your arms wide out to each side, with the elbows bent enough so that the position feels**

powerful in the arms as well as in the belly. (What you are doing here is bringing the power in your arms and hands into harmony with your belly muscles, and your knee muscles as well.)

4. Finally, move your arms back to the beginning position, in front of you, arms somewhat bent, elbows down and in. Do this basic "up-down-out-in" movement several times, but quit before you become tired. Give one breath to each movement, as seems best for you. And remember that your goal is to tighten and activate the abdominal muscles powerfully and yet pleasurably in each position.

BELLY WAKE-UPS

Now for yet another way to wake up different muscles in the belly region, stand quietly a moment with your balance on both feet equally. Breathe.

Then bring your arms forward as you raise one leg in front of you also, balancing on the other leg. Breathe into this position for a full breath cycle. Then bring both your arms and your raised leg behind you as you bend forward to keep your balance. Hold this position for one breath, activating your belly muscles to maintain the posture. Return to the forward position for a breath, and then go back to the back position

again for another breath. Then just relax, standing on both feet, and notice how you are feeling in your belly region after this powerful activation movement.

Now stand on the other foot, and do the same movements, forward and then backward, with the other leg in the air, a couple of times. Then stand quietly, eyes closed, and tune in to the rushes of energy through your body, which were activated by this simple yet dynamic movement. Try it for yourself now.

⊙

With these five basic belly-activation postures, you have the beginning of a movement routine that takes only five minutes or so from your busy sedentary day and that can make all the difference in the world to your belly condition. Your challenge is this: See if you can get to know these five postures and movements by heart, through spending time with this book, until you can do them on your own.

This is the second basic program I have outlined for you. I am giving you the tools. You do what you want to with them. You should certainly feel free to come up with your own variations on the general theme of holding postures that activate your belly muscles. There are literally thousands of such postures, and I have given you the first five.

During the rest of your life, I challenge you to discover the rest of them!

I will also be writing, in chapter 11, about helping machines that you can use to even more powerfully activate your belly region. But I feel it is always important to devise a routine that is at least 50 percent based on movements and postures that require no special equipment. So what you have learned in this chapter should stand as an introduction to an entire universe of movements and positions that you can do, on your own anywhere, to immediately bring you more in touch with the beautiful warrior spirit in your belly.

You might want to go back right now and read through the five postures/movements again, even do them again, so that you begin the process of learning them by heart.

8

Emotional and Sexual Considerations

I've been very interested, and sometimes amused, to talk with therapists of different traditions about their interpretation of a man with a belly. As you perhaps know, there are three classic schools of therapy in the Western world, and each of these traditions has its separate notion about how to approach the belly question. Let me give you these different approaches, and you can see which of them rings truest for your own condition.

First of all, in the tradition of Sigmund Freud, a big belly is often seen as a manifestation of what is called an oral fixation. Babies begin life with a strong fixation on sucking and eating, of course. And associated with this urgent desire to suck is a great pleasure in the actual act of sucking.

As babies mature into two- and three-year-olds, they usually go through a phase during which the oral fixation shifts to the proverbial anal fixation, toilet training is the key issue, and sensual pleasures become associated with the anal and genital regions, and with the body as a whole, in action.

Many children, however, for complex reasons, remain somewhat stuck in the oral phase of their development. Basically, these children hold on to a relationship with their mothers that should be mostly let go of—the early intimate, nursing relationship. Sometimes a mother instigates this fixation by hungering herself for a continuation of this intimacy, especially if she is not getting such intimacy from her husband/partner. At other times just the opposite can happen. A sudden end of the nursing relationship, before the infant is ready to let go of this first phase of relating, can leave the child caught in a prolonged yearning for what was lost too soon.

In either case, according to the Freudian understanding, the fixation on the oral stage will manifest itself later on in life through such habits as compulsive overeating and drinking, and a general tendency to regress to infantile feelings and body condition. I am sure you have known grown men who have soft, pudgy bodies that reminded you of an overgrown baby. Often their voices remain high, and they express an emotional immaturity as well. These qualities are not necessarily negative, by the way. Most of us love babies, so we can enjoy being around a man who is a big baby.

The belly region in such a man will of course be weak and overextended. And because the state of being a helpless baby has so many positive aspects, it is often almost impossible for such a man to choose to let go of its advantages just to get rid of the belly that goes along with the condition. In fact, the belly represents the positive as well as the negative aspects of such a personality.

In Freudian analysis, the approach to such a supposedly neurotic personality is to let the client go back and relive early childhood experiences, in the hope that through seeing the roots of the fixation, he will come to growth and maturation. There is really no focus on movement in such classical analysis, so even though insights might come to a person in therapy of this sort, he would not necessarily experience much change in the belly muscles.

Now let's consider the tradition of Wilhelm Reich, whose therapy techniques evoke a powerful opportunity for personality growth and physical transformations. The bioenergetic school of therapy developed by Reich's student Alexander Lowen, and the radix school of Charles Kelley, also a student of Reich, offer quite a different insight from Freud's into how to approach a man and his belly.

When Freud looked at a client's belly he most likely saw images of the client's past. But when

Reich looked at a client's belly he almost certainly saw blocked energy flows in the client's body in the present moment.

For Reich there were definite bands of tension up and down the body, corresponding to inner energy centers that could be either open and free flowing with their energy exchange or blocked and inhibited. It is, of course, quite curious to notice that most men with bellies have a definite band around their midriffs below which there is little or no fat, and above which exists a belt of fat and weakness.

Reich felt, to put it very simply, that a man with a belly is inhibiting the flow of sexual excitation that would normally flow up and down the body. If this flow was open and free, there would be no blocking of energy in the belly. There would also be no fat accumulation and no muscular weakness in the belly region.

Reich would agree in principle with what Freud said about infantile fixation, but he would expand this quickly to include difficulties in the next phase of a child's development, mainly in the relationship between father and son, and the extent to which the father allows the son to stand up and feel his personal power in his father's presence. Reich would also mention the importance of a father allowing his son to have sexual feelings toward his mother during the early years of his life. According to Reich, any inhibition of the child's natural sexual feelings would lead to problems in his belly later on in life if the inhibitions continued.

To treat this problem of blocked energy flow, Reich would prescribe sessions that would directly stimulate the discharge of the client's early inhibitions and anxieties, so that the flow of excitation and power could be finally opened up in the client's body in the present moment.

Alexander Lowen took this approach further by designing actual movements and stress postures that would stimulate the flow of energy through the belly region. The exercises I taught you in the last chapter are variations on the general themes that Lowen developed.

There is a third major therapy tradition that we should look to in this light. Carl Jung took quite a different approach to working with a man with a big belly. Jung focused primarily on the symbolic nature of consciousness, delving into spiritual and mystical realms that Freud and Reich tended to avoid. For Jung, a big belly was representative of a special feeling deep within a client's psychic structure, quite similar to that of James Joyce's character Bloom, whom I mentioned at the beginning of our discussion. The human mind has a vast potential for symbolic associations, of course, and Jung would encourage a client to accept these associations completely and actively indulge in exploring dreams and fantasies that would shed deeper light on his belly itself. Whereas Freud was focused on getting clients "back to normal," Jung was more accepting of each person's existing condition, seeing spiritual significance instead of neurosis in most deviations from the cultural norm.

I know that I have given a terribly oversimplified sketch of these complex geniuses and their feelings about the belly question, but my intent has only been to show that there are three different approaches, and that for me all these approaches are important to consider if you want to come to a deeper appreciation of your own belly.

⊙

Can you feel all three of these aspects in terms of your relationship with your belly: big baby oral fixation, blocked sexual and personal-power energy flows in your body, and symbolic meaning to your belly?

⊙

In my opinion, one of the main emotional aspects of a big belly has to do with early childhood feelings of sadness and lack of adequate attention and love. I spent a couple of years in my early twenties working as a social psychologist at a preschool. Some of these children I worked with already had the basic posture that would lead to a big belly condition in adult life.

Suffering from deep feelings of rejection by their parents, they became stuck in a pouting posture. Reich and Lowen have spoken much about this feeling. The child first of all feels angry at not getting enough attention. But the release of this anger at the parents only results in punishment and further rejection. So the child learns to block the flow of anger, and instead stands around pouting, with an extended lower lip and a big belly.

Such early blocking of anger is common in many of us, of course. And I would venture to say that perhaps the majority of men with bellies have this blocking as at least a part of their adult condition. A child seeks gratification. First this gratification comes through sucking. Then it should generalize into receiving adequate amounts of love and, of course, satisfying nutrition as well. But when the love is somehow not adequate, the child will often fixate on eating as a means of satisfying frustrated needs on other levels (love).

⊙

Did you get enough love as a child, or were you one of those kids who pouted and carried around blocked anger in your belly? Give yourself some time to put this book aside if you want to right now, and breathe into whatever memories or insights come to you.

⊙

Young men tend to have hard bellies during the period in which they are wild young warriors out hunting sexual gratification. To be single and hunting sexual fulfillment can be both exciting and anxiety provoking. And both these emotional conditions tend to burn a lot of calories.

But when a man finds a person with whom to settle down, a relaxation usually comes into the man's entire nature, and with this relaxation comes a tendency to put on some weight. As humans we have a tendency to overemphasize our hunger for security. And when we get the security we seek, we tend to sink into a reduced level of activity. And often with this loss of vitality comes the big belly syndrome.

How can such a condition be reversed? Some men go out and start chasing young girls in an attempt to regain the old warrior spirit. Others take on risky business ventures to activate the adrenaline rush of earlier days. Others say to hell with the flat belly and just relax into a lifetime of the easy life.

⊙

What is your story? Pause and look back on the progression of your life. Where has it taken you, and where would you like to go from here?

⊙

There is, of course, a direct link between sexual power and personal power. If you are afraid to express yourself sexually, you will tend to block the flow of energy through your belly and genitals. The result will be general weakness.

⊙

What were you like as a teenager in this regard? Were you inhibited sexually, somehow guilty about your wild wet-dream fantasies? And how did your sexual inhibitions affect the muscles of your belly? Look back and see what comes to mind as you remember your sexual feelings when you were a teenager.

And now, in the present, is your sexual energy free to flow, or is there still an inhibition down there, a denial of your desires, a fear of activating your sexual powers? What experience comes to you if you put this book aside for a few moments, put one hand over your genitals and one over your belly, close your eyes, and see if you can feel a dynamic interaction between these two regions of your body?

⊙

Such a meditation is highly recommended as a regular reflection on your sexual and power centers. The belly is of course supposed to be the center of your personal power. If you are well grounded in your personal power, there will be a good flow of energy all the way from the bottoms of your feet, up your legs, through your genital region, and into your belly.

⊙

Close your eyes and see if you can be aware of your feet, your legs, your genitals, and your belly, all at the same time, as you breathe the next few breaths.

And finally, while you are aware of the lower regions of your body, allow your awareness to expand to your heart, your throat and mouth, and see what emotions you find deep down in your genitals, belly, and heart that might want to come up and out, be released right now.

⊙

When the pouting, frustrated, unhappy child finally releases the feelings inside, very often the child cries. I remember over and over again seeing a child with a big belly and a pouting lower lip on the playground or in the classroom where I was working, and asking this child to come into my room for a moment. The child would stand there with totally blocked feelings inside, and then, step by step, if I did my role well, he or she would finally release those feelings, and the big, weak belly would suddenly be transformed into a powerful, flat belly, either through spasms of crying or through the release of shouting and aggressive action.

Crying itself should be considered actively as a belly exercise. There is really nothing better for the belly than crying. Watch any infant as it cries. The belly muscles contract with bravado power— crying is an aggressive act, after all. Screaming requires powerful contractions of the belly muscles, and the hitting and kicking that accompany crying activate the belly muscles as well.

So I put out to you this possibility. Maybe your belly is weak and big because you have for most of your life been inhibiting your need to express your sorrows and frustrations through crying. What do you think?

Having been raised on cattle ranches, I was, of course, not supposed to break down and cry; this was the ultimate disgrace for a little cowboy. And still now, as an adult who has had plenty of growthful therapy sessions and who considers himself quite open and free with his emotions, I know I am a little blocked with my expression of sorrow. Even today I can recall those old-time belly feelings of holding back the tears, standing with a big belly and completely blocked feelings in front of the cowhands and my brothers.

⊙

There are two basic childhood expressions that seem to be caught up in grown-up men's bellies. The first is this: "Poor me, nobody loves me, I'm all alone and I just want to cry!" Try saying these words three or four times, and see how the words affect your feelings and your belly.

The other side of this coin is this: "I hate you, I hate everybody!" Try saying these words over quite a few times now, and see how they awaken old feelings.

As a great challenge, let me leave you with this suggestion: Regularly look to see what emotions you are holding in your belly that would like to come out. Let them say what they want to say, and let the discharges come as often as possible. Right now, pause and open yourself up to the experience of whatever feelings you find under pressure inside you.

9

Discipline Versus Self-Love

Psychological theories can help in our general understanding of our relationship with our bellies, but, ultimately, action is required to generate change in the body, as I have mentioned already. A weak belly almost always is an indication of a lack of discipline somewhere in the personality. And if you want to reverse this situation, you are going to have to develop an increased sense of discipline.

What is your relationship with the very concept of self-discipline?

Babies and young children are noted for their lack of self-discipline. This is an ability that develops later on in childhood. And, as I mentioned in the last chapter, many men with bellies are caught to one extent or another in infantile tendencies toward undisciplined indulging. So it is a great step for many men, especially at the levels of eating and drinking, to develop a newfound sense of discipline with which to control consumption habits.

The same is true of movement habits. If you are habitually lazy with regard to muscular activity, if you like to just slouch around with a loose, undisciplined body, then it can be quite a step to shift out of these habits into a more active self-image.

What are some realistic steps that can aid in the long-term development of increased discipline?

First of all, it is important to see the purpose behind disciplined behavior. In this regard, the recent development of the therapy tradition of behavioral psychology can shed valuable light on weight reduction and muscle toning. According to behavioral psychologists, if you want to change a habit, you need to understand the rewards you will receive when you discipline yourself in the desired direction, and you need to understand the punishments that can come if you fail in your discipline routines. Behaviorism is based on the primal human fact that we naturally gravitate toward positive rewards and avoid negative punishments.

⊙

What will you gain if you discipline yourself to eat a healthier diet and increase your movement routines, for instance? Here is a list of possible gains; check the ones that would come to you if you increased your sense of self-discipline.

1. Healthier body ____
2. Better love life ____
3. More enjoyable self-image ____
4. More personal power ____
5. More success at work ____
6. Lighter feeling in the body ____
7. Better social acceptance ____
8. Reduced restaurant/food bills ____
9. Emotional growth and enjoyment ____
10. Transformation of life-style ____

There are, of course, many more specific rewards that can come to you if you discipline yourself into a belly condition that you prefer. Make your own list if you think of other pleasures that would come your way if you reduced your belly size and increased your muscle tone.

In the other direction, you should consider a list of negative aspects of having a big belly, and what might happen if you fail to discipline yourself.

1. Bad feelings in the body ____
2. Loss of sexual attractiveness ____

3. **Weakness and failure in physical encounters** ____
4. **Bad social image** ____
5. **Limited success at work** ____
6. **Danger of colon cancer and other health problems** ____
7. **Blocked emotions** ____
8. **Sense of personal failure** ____
9. **Rejection by loved ones** ____
10. **General sluggishness of consciousness** ____

Add to this general list your own personal list of problems associated with failing to lose your big belly.

Overall, when you look at the pros and cons of weight loss and belly transformation, is it worth the effort to push yourself into a disciplined routine at this point in your life? Is there actually enough to be gained to provoke you into action? Stop and honestly assess your present feelings.

⊙

If you do feel that you are motivated by the rewards and punishments involved, then how can you turn this motivational energy into disciplined action?

The trick lies in the nature of habit alteration,

as I have suggested. You need to choose a simple step that you are fairly confident you can make, and test yourself with that step. Perhaps you have already begun this process with one or more of the steps I have suggested in previous chapters. Just doing the abdominal exhale once an hour is one of the best steps, because it involves the remembering process itself. If you simply never think about your belly, you are not going to be able to discipline yourself to do anything to its advantage. So remembering to do something, even something remarkably simple and enjoyable, is the first step, the step of consciousness itself.

Then you can begin adding other steps that you are fairly confident about succeeding with. And each time you act, you will want to reflect on the rewards and punishments associated with your challenge of belly transformation.

Discipline itself involves four ingredients. First of all, you must discipline your mind to remember to set aside time and energy to act. Then you must have a clear notion of what the necessary actions are. Then you must actually move yourself through the actions, be they physical movements, altered eating patterns, or inner meditations. Finally, you must regularly reflect on how your actions are affecting your life, so that you tune in to the rewards that come from your actions.

The words that outline this discipline process should be written out clearly at this point:

Remembering
Understanding
Acting
Reflecting

If you approach discipline in this spirit, you can also include the other vital element of our program: self-love. For long-term success and enjoyment of a discipline routine, self-love is essential. By *self-love* I mean that you act with the conscious intention of giving yourself something that will make you happy. So with each disciplined action that you make, it is important to consciously explore the pleasures that come through the action. With this approach, you can quickly transform an act of discipline into an act of desire.

⊙

Reflect on each of the following dimensions I have offered thus far for transforming your belly, and see if you can find pleasure in the disciplined routines:

1. **Memory expeditions**
2. **Emotional reflections and release**
3. **Movements and stress positions**

4. Self-image meditations
5. Improvement of eating habits

⊙

It does require mental discipline to make the effort to do each of these actions. But there is also pleasure awaiting you in the very act, as well as in the final payoff.

My experience in giving people exercises and meditations to do at home is this: If there isn't an immediate gratification available in the movement or meditation, people just won't do what I recommend, even if they know that down the road there could be a positive reward.

So with this reality in mind, I have done my best to come up with suggestions that are always a pleasure to do once you understand how to go into them properly. And let me be honest with you—I prefer immediate gratification as well for any program I discipline myself to do.

So look to include pleasure and self-love in your acts of discipline if you want to succeed in anything. If you love your discipline, discipline will love you too.

10

Wisdom of the Belly

Imagine waking up tomorrow morning and going about your day without bothering to have anything for breakfast. Perhaps you have a cup of tea or some juice, but imagine not eating your customary food in the morning. What would happen to you? Most likely some part of you would panic at the very thought, even while another part of you would praise the act as a fine step in disciplining yourself toward a smaller belly.

All of us do in fact fear the experience of going hungry. We have a powerful conditioned appetite, which serves to regulate our food intake. And, unfortunately, this appetite control center in our brains is almost always somewhat out of touch with the reality of our nutritional needs.

For instance, when you wake up tomorrow morning, you will in fact already be in possession of enough inner stores of calories to run your body quite satisfactorily for at least a week or two, with no nutritional problem at all. Most of you could go a month eating hardly anything and do very well, once you adjusted to the fasting routine.

But regardless of your realistic supplies of inner food reserves, your psychological reaction to missing breakfast would probably be traumatic. You would feel hungry first of all, with your appetite anticipating your regular breakfast but not getting it. Anticipation is nine-tenths of the story when it comes to hunger, as I am sure you know from experience. Thoughts about what you are going to eat next in life are the prime motivation for pushing you into a hungry state so that you seek out what you have been thinking about.

So discipline in altering your eating habits is mostly a matter of old thought habits fighting against new thoughts, which crazy books like this provoke you into thinking. When you combine your old thought patterns with the first pangs of emptiness in your stomach, you encounter a force so powerful that most of us are overcome by the hunger pangs.

What I suggest first of all in making some headway against your old overeating habits is this: Just start to observe the process of hunger and appetite in action during the next few days. Get up tomorrow morning with the intention of perhaps not eating breakfast, for instance. As the minutes tick by when you would normally have been eating breakfast, observe closely what happens to your thoughts, your emotions, and your feelings in your stomach. To see your automatic feeding-time mechanism in action is a great step toward gaining some control over this compulsive behavior, if you in fact want to gain such control.

And when you do surrender to this urge to eat something, watch what happens as you eat what you want to eat. How fast does the hunger urge go away, for instance? And how long do you remain free of appetite, before it again rises to the surface of your consciousness to push you toward your next meal?

What is wrong with being empty? Why do we try to keep ourselves stuffed with food so as to avoid the empty-stomach feeling completely?

Certainly old Sigmund could have given us some convincing arguments regarding early feeding habits as infants, and the instinctive programming of human beings to keep as full as possible so as not to starve to death. We are, in fact, creatures of animal programmings when it comes to eating, and these programmings certainly made much sense a few thousand years ago, when it was important to put on a little fat in the summer and autumn months because the winters could be long and hungry indeed.

But all this has changed for most of us in Western civilization. Our problem is just the opposite.

We have so much food available that we endanger ourselves through overeating and almost never face any real danger of starvation from lack of food.

Specific statistics vary in degree, but there is definite evidence that the average man in our society carries 2 to 5 pounds of extremely noxious muck inside his intestinal tract. This gooey gluck sticks to the sides of the intestines and seriously interferes with their normal absorption processes. The stuff is made up mostly of half-digested mucous foods, such as dairy products (especially cheese), pork and beef fat (especially fried fat), and, to a lesser extent, other meat products.

Some men pack around 10 or even 15 pounds of added muck in their intestines. This is a serious condition, because diseases such as cancer of the colon are directly related to this constant irritation. Furthermore, this muck definitely interferes with a person's digestion process on a regular basis, leaving one feeling chronically sluggish, polluted, and poisoned.

Is this you? If so, what can you do about it, and why did you get yourself into this condition in the first place?

⊙

Take some time to reflect on the condition of your intestines—are they habitually too empty or too full?

⊙

One definite treatment for a clogged-up intestinal tract is to get your doctor to prescribe several professional colonic treatments, in which water or wheat-grass juice or some other decongestant liquid is pumped up your behind under pressure, all the way through your colon, then through your large intestine, and then is allowed to come back out the tube with everything it has picked up from the intestinal lining in the process. This is an amazing experience, because usually you can watch the water before it goes into you through a clear tube and see its pureness, and then you can watch it coming out a few minutes later, and actually see the terrible stuff that you have had inside you literally for years on end. It is a horror show to watch going by, but it is a blessing to have out of you.

This colonic treatment is actually quite painless, because you get to control the rate of flow of water into you, and the pressure as well, so you never overextend your comfort zone. I wonder why doctors don't prescribe this treatment on a regular basis for about half of their men patients, to tell you the truth. The cost is not great, and I recommend that you have two or three treatments, within a couple of weeks, to really clean your bowels thoroughly.

There is, of course, a catch to this treatment,

and it is this: Most men are quite honestly afraid and embarrassed to go and have the treatment. Nobody likes the idea of having a tube stuck up his behind (although it only goes a couple of inches and doesn't hurt at all), and no self-respecting man wants to admit that he's full of, you know—literally—shit.

But I challenge you to overcome this resistance, and to get yourself a colonic treatment. Give yourself one for your next birthday. I know most of you won't, but I wish most of you would. The colonic machine deserves more praise and usage than it gets.

That is one way to help your bowels and intestines get empty for a new start in life. But you can also approach the question from the other end of your digestive tract, and stop eating so many mucous foods (basically dairy and meat and refined flour products). Add to this regular exercise, which will bounce your intestines around enough to help dislodge some of the crud in your system, and you are making another step. And, at deeper levels, begin to meditate on the wisdom and beauty of emptiness.

This is actually the last major notion I want to leave with you: the wisdom and beauty of being empty. We are a culture that has an absolutely terrible relationship with emptiness. We are compulsively seeking to be full all the time, without even bothering to check on the quality of what we are stuffing ourselves with. All you have to do is watch television for an evening to see that we have reached an all-time low in the quality of what we put into us. Whether it be sensory inputs or edible inputs, we constantly fill ourselves up with whatever might be available, rather than enjoying the kinds of experiences that silence and an empty stomach can bring us.

Along with psychological and medical influences, I have been very much influenced by the spiritual tradition of the Zen heritage from China and Japan, wherein fullness is always balanced with emptiness for optimum health and a good life. To deeply experience the wonderful tastes of a good meal, it is first necessary to be empty of food long enough that the contrast is appreciated. Furthermore, rather than running away from the threat of starvation through overeating all the time, it is best, according to the Zen teachers, to face the experience of hunger head on, so that the fear can be let go of and a realistic sense of appetite finally gained in one's lifetime.

⊙

What is your relationship with hunger and emptiness?

11

Machines That Help

The human body moving freely can bring about quite a bit of rapid transformation in muscle tone and strength. Calories are burnt rapidly, especially with aerobic exercise that really gets the heart pounding. And one's self-image gets a big boost; one sees oneself in a new, healthier light.

But the human body is also designed to interact with the surrounding environment. In the old days, a man often carried something in his hand for protection, for instance, and this weapon's weight stimulated a regular added contraction in the belly muscles. Most work involved the manipulation of objects, which in turn exercised the muscles of the abdomen.

These days, however, we don't carry weapons.

Most of us don't even own one, nor know how to use one. So the basic warrior experience of wielding something in one's hands has been lost, unless we consciously act to regain this dimension of human life.

Also, for a great many of us, our daily work is done not with the belly muscles but with our mental muscles. I know most of my work involves either just sitting here pounding on these keys, which requires almost zero bellywork, or sitting with a client exercising my ear muscles more than anything else. I've been lucky as a therapist in that I almost always combine movements with talking therapy and do the movements with my clients, so there is some action in my work. I even do a lot of martial arts mock fighting with clients, which awakens my warrior spirit along with that of my clients when we do it together. But still, when I think back to younger days of cowboy work, and to times when I have worked as a carpenter as a break from therapy work, I realize that I lead a basically sedentary life when it comes to working with my hands in the environment. What about you?

To compensate for this lack in physical exertion, there are a number of really wonderful machines you can get these days, if you want to increase your belly action beyond what you encounter through movement. Some of these machines are complex and expensive, but some of them are inexpensive, or even free. Let me survey some of those that I consider personally valuable and enjoyable to use, and you can see if you want to get one or more of them for your own use.

First and perhaps foremost, there are simple hand weights, which you can buy for ten or twenty dollars. These are wonderful for daily exercise routines. I prefer the ones that are metal weights covered in plastic, so you don't hurt yourself and so the metal isn't directly visible. I use weights that are 3.5 kilograms, or 7.7 pounds each, and I think this is a reasonable weight for an average-sized man.

When you first get the weights in your hands, they might seem a little heavy if you haven't been using weights for a while or doing heavy work with your arm muscles. But quickly you will build adequate muscles for using them creatively.

These are simple weights that you hold in each hand and move in ways that accentuate muscle tension throughout the body. I believe that human beings have an actual genetic predisposition to have something of this basic weight in their hands, and I hope that you can tap into the magical power that rises up in the body when you are working with these weights.

Working is not the right word. You will really enjoy the playful feeling you get when you tap into your power to swing and hold and move these weights around your body. When I think of all the "machines" I am going to talk about in this chapter, these weights stand as primary in my recommendation to you, if you want some instant acceleration in your muscle power development and your general powerful self-image.

One way to use these weights is this: Stand with your feet fairly wide apart, and then begin very gently exploring what happens when you move the weights into a position, and then hold them in that position while you breathe into the stress created throughout your body. At first your belly muscles might not even go to work at all. But then you will make a connection between your mind and your belly, and suddenly power will flow into the abdominal muscles to compensate for the stress the weights are causing.

In essence, the stress of the weights will wake up muscles that otherwise lie dormant. And this wakening of muscles is such a pleasure to experience—it's like coming alive again as a man of power!

There are three basic things you can do with hand weights. You can hold them in at least a thousand stress positions, each of which is a spiritual meditation in itself. You can also make slow, swinging movements through the air around you with the weights, breathing in rhythmic ways to establish a ritual pattern that combines breath and movement. And, third, you can advance into spontaneous movements that take you into a dance with the weights. Music can add an important dimension to this free-form workout.

If you don't want to buy weights, you can play

with a large stone in similar ways, or take just about anything of reasonable weight and do movement routines with it and your arms.

For instance, you can take a stick or club in your hands and swing it in definite ways around your head and body, like a samurai warrior, and tap into a beautiful rush of power in your body. You can also buy a ceremonial wooden sword from almost any martial arts center and explore movements on your own, or join up and take some lessons if you want to. But you want to be careful that you don't get into an overly macho martial arts training program, which loses much of the playful spirit we have been talking about. Getting too hard is for me as unhealthy as getting too soft in the belly. But you can be your own guide when you look into such programs. Or you can just buy a wooden sword, of about a yard or meter in length, and develop your own spontaneous movements with it. Like I said, a stick from the woods can serve you almost as well.

Of course, playing tennis or squash is also excellent for the belly muscles, as is basketball or soccer or volleyball. To join an easygoing weekly local club in a sport is highly advisable for belly transformations, as long as you get yourself in reasonable shape before going out onto the field.

In terms of more complicated machines for belly fitness, there is, first of all, the basic exercise bench that you can buy for one to two hundred dollars, on which you do sit-ups with your knees bent and feet anchored. This is fine, but if you want to spend the money for a machine to help with your belly, perhaps you should go one step further and get what I consider the ultimate fitness machine for the belly—the rowing machine. It gives you a feeling of movement that is deeply meditative and works the entire body perfectly. Especially during the winter months, when it might be too cold to go running regularly, the rowing machine is just terrific, an ode to technology.

Some people are crazy about their cross-country skiing machines as well, and you should try one to see if this particular movement feels better than that of the rowing machine. Certainly for fitness, the cross-country skiing machine is tops, although I personally prefer the experience of rowing.

There are many other exercise machines of similar bent. All of them have the value of providing resistance to your muscles, to increase the workout value per minute. My only restrictive suggestion would be that you avoid too much heavy weight lifting, which develops brute lifting power but often constricts your potential for spontaneous movements.

So I encourage you in general to begin to seek out your favorite helper machine for transforming your belly. Take your time in this search, see what is available, perhaps use a friend's machine before buying your own. And *please*, always hold in mind that machine-aided exercise should never be more than half of your overall workout routine. Free movement is still the foundation to a healthy integration of mind and body.

I also recommend slow stretching as important to a well-rounded program. Hatha yoga (physical stretching) stands as the classic champion in helping one understand movement, teaching a deep relationship between muscles and consciousness. I strongly recommend balancing a program using exercise machines with a weekly class in hatha yoga.

Obviously there are many paths you can explore in searching for what satisfies you most in movement programs. Some people take care of their bellies through just dancing regularly. Dance is one of the oldest and most powerful ways of keeping healthy while you explore your creative expression through movement. Going somewhere to dance once a week can be one of the most pleasurable disciplines you will ever find.

To aid in choosing a movement program, make a list of ways you can bring regular concentrated exercise into your weekly schedule.

Good luck in hunting down your favorite means of exercising your belly muscles!

12

Belly Consciousness

We have covered quite a lot of important ground regarding your relationship with your belly. On five
different dimensions, you now have practical steps
you can make if you want to improve your belly condition. Perhaps the most important basic notion
we have been approaching from several directions
thus far is this idea of permanently expanding your
moment-to-moment awareness of your belly region
while you go about your daily routines.

**How much of each day would you estimate that
you are aware of your belly feelings? Are you**

mostly unconscious of what is going on down there, or are you alert to the changes in muscle tone, emotional flows, and other more subtle feelings that are regularly happening in that region?

⊙

The physiological and emotional reality is this: At any given moment, throughout your entire life, there is something dynamic happening down in your belly region. There is always one emotion or another present in the belly for you to tune in to, and your belly is therefore your constant barometer of what is happening deep down in your psyche.

When I am talking with a client during therapy sessions, I very often, perhaps ten times a session, suggest that the client notice how the discussion is affecting the feelings in his or her belly region. After a few sessions with a client, all I have to do is look down at a person's belly, and it is understood that I am asking for a focusing on the belly experience at that moment.

The greatest challenge of all in life, of course, is to become more conscious of what is happening inside you and around you at any given moment. And because the belly is really the seat of the emotions, belly awareness is one of the primary vehicles for encouraging expanded consciousness.

The curious thing about belly consciousness is that you can increase your physiological awareness, your emotional awareness, and your deeper intuitive and spiritual awareness all in the same simple act of focusing your consciousness on the belly region.

If belly consciousness is so important, and also simple to experience regularly, why is it that most people go around almost totally unaware of the great symphony of experiences happening down in their belly regions?

The answer is straightforward, but sometimes difficult to do anything about. Most people are somewhat afraid of some of their deeper emotions. They avoid feeling painful emotions, for instance. And they run away from emotions that are associated with fear. They also avoid making contact with their inner feelings of repulsion and disgust. In a word, all the negative feelings that naturally rise up in the belly as a reaction to encounters with the outside world are habitually blocked from rising up to consciousness. Almost all of us have these automatic habits of avoiding negative feelings. And, unfortunately for our overall emotional health, we do have the ability to automatically push our feelings down into the belly and ignore them completely.

Do you do this sometimes?

And if you do, what is the result?

Both in my own life and in nearly too much

work as a therapist, I have found over and over again that emotions that were ignored and pushed down to be hidden and buried in the belly region can live there literally for a lifetime, carrying their negative charge and disturbing the deeper emotional processes as well as chronically upsetting one's digestion and belly fitness. Buried emotions are not lost. We fool ourselves if we think we can just ignore a bad feeling and make it go away permanently.

Often I have found that men with big bellies have tried to bury their rejected feelings under as big a layer of fat as possible, just as we think we can bury our atomic waste deep enough that it will never rise and hurt us. I think in both cases we are seriously fooling ourselves. With buried belly feelings, I know this is true. And I also know that the only way to permanently get rid of old feelings is to let them rise to the surface, be experienced and accepted, and then be let go of.

The main way of encouraging this healing process in the belly is simply to reestablish an open, honest communication channel between your conscious mind and your belly feelings. I have given you quite a number of approaches to this ultimate goal. The choice, of course, as I said in the beginning, is up to you. Most people go through life without directly acting to heal their belly zones, so you can be assured you are among the majority if you choose to put this book on the shelf and carry on with your present belly condition. But, on the other hand, it is so simple to go in the opposite direction that I hope you do make a step toward treating your belly with the kind of love that heals.

Final Words/
A Lifetime Fitness Plan

Now that you have read through the various programs and suggestions of this book, the question arises: What in fact are you going to do, or not going to do, to expand your relationship with your belly and bring about positive change where you desire it?

The first step is always to go back and read through the bold-type exercise and contemplation sections of the text, as often as needed to learn the programs by heart, so you can do them on a somewhat regular basis if you want to.

A next important step is to make a list of what you want to focus on in the next few weeks, so that you have in hand a clear written outline of your objectives regarding your belly condition.

Some of you will find these two suggestions adequate for your growth process, as you use this book as your guide for doing the exercises and meditations. Some of you, however, might find that, with just you and the book, motivation gets lost very easily. If this is the case, let me suggest some additional ways in which you can encourage yourself to focus regularly on programs that will enhance your relationship with your belly.

WORKING WITH A FRIEND

Often it is very helpful to seek out someone with similar interests to yours when you are trying to succeed with a new program or challenge. Ideally you might find or form a men's belly group in your community, using this book as a basic manual to stimulate your interaction. Such a support group can prove invaluable, and I strongly recommend it.

You can also get together with just one friend who has read this book or a similar discussion and help each other to explore the various exercises and meditations. This is especially helpful when doing the guided memory and insight meditations. Many people find it hard to have to read the book, then close their eyes and do a meditation, then open their eyes and read another suggestion, then close their eyes and do that meditation, and so on and so forth, moving from leader to experiencer over and over again.

And here we come to a point of great importance, which emerges out of the wisdom of the therapy relationship. Growth is stimulated quite powerfully when there is one person taking the role of guide or leader while the other person takes the role of experiencer for a certain period of time.

In my therapy work I of course use my voice as the main stimulant for guiding a client in a growth process. When a client can relax, close his eyes, and simply take in a spoken suggestion to act upon, then an ideal situation for deep experiencing is created.

I have given you many of the same suggestions in this book that I use with clients on a regular basis when doing bellywork. So if you are working with a friend, one of you can read a particular suggestion from the book, or paraphrase it however you want, while the other relaxes with eyes closed, takes in the suggestion, and goes deeply into whatever new experience is stimulated by the suggestion.

Then, after a couple of minutes of relaxed quiet, the friend acting as guide reads a new suggestion, so that the experiencer has an effortless new direction to move in.

You can spend half an hour going through particular sections of the book in this way. Then you can switch roles either at that point or later on in the day or week, and lead your friend through the same experience you were led through.

This is one of the finest ways to grow, as you

take advantage of professional suggestions while sharing your inner experiences with a friend after a session. Such mutual support will accelerate the growth process. And you will find that you can enter quite a mature evolutionary process by carrying on in whatever directions the two of you naturally choose to explore together.

Your friend does not have to have a "belly problem" to guide you, by the way. You can ask anyone to play the role of guide and benefit considerably. You can also get out a tape recorder and record the suggestions from the book yourself, then play back your recording while you relax and take in the suggestions.

GUIDED SESSIONS

Another avenue for support in your exploration of your relationship with your belly is to use the taped guided sessions which I have prepared on this subject, and which I also regularly give to clients to take home and use during the week between sessions. For many years I have been using this medium for offering clients additional guidance at home, and my experience has been that a great amount of insight and emotional growth can occur through such cassette-program guidance in one's home environment. Certain people need direct interaction with a therapist or other helper in order to grow, but the majority of us can in fact help ourselves on our own, if we have the proper guidance tools. The available cassettes are listed in the final pages of the book.

WHERE YOU STAND NOW—BELLY-WISE

One thing is for certain—you are going to be in an intimate relationship with your belly for the rest of your life. So it makes sense to consciously enhance this vital relationship on a regular basis. Let's take a quick overview of the various ways you have learned in this book for tuning in to your belly region and encouraging health, fitness, and good feelings down there.

We begin our discussion by looking at four factors that determine your belly shape and health. First of all, there is the actual size and performance of your stomach and intestines, determined by the food you eat on a regular basis. Second, there is the muscle tone that you maintain or fail to maintain in your abdominal muscles. Third, there is the emotional flow or lack of it through the belly region. And, finally, there is the cognitive self-image, which underlies all the other influences on your belly size and health.

$\odot$

As a final suggestion in this program, let me recommend the most vital belly contemplation you can do each and every day, if you really want to

optimize your relationship with your midriff. When you wake up each morning, begin to develop the habit of sitting on the edge of the bed for just a few moments before getting up, or at some point before leaving the bedroom. Quietly turn your attention to your breathing, then to your whole body's presence in the room as you breathe. Then tune in to your belly and say good morning to your midriff. Make conscious contact with this region of your body before you get in gear for the day. Greet your belly like a friend in the morning. Feel a flow of love down into this region. Provide the conscious, positive spark of involvement with your belly that will stimulate a full day of belly awareness and action to improve your belly condition.

I have emphasized that the key element in belly transformation is an ongoing awareness of your belly as you go through each and every day. This vital link between your mind and your belly is in fact what brings about transformation.

So as you sit there in the morning doing your belly contemplation for a few moments, first of all make intimate contact with this region of your body, both as a physical and also as an emotional presence. And then have a little morning talk with your belly, telling it what you are going to do for the both of you through the day to improve its condition.

At this point in your morning contemplation, run through your mind the four factors that you can act on to improve your midriff's shape and health:

THE FOOD YOU EAT. **Tell your belly what you are going to do to eat less food, and healthier food, in a more relaxed digestive manner. Commit yourself to a small step in the right direction, by agreeing to cut out one dessert, for instance, or even cutting out one meal, or one candy bar, or one glass of wine or beer. Make one definite commitment, and see if you can hold it in your mind all day, and stick to it.**

THE MOVEMENTS YOU MAKE. **Commit yourself first of all to being as aware as you can of all the movements you make during the day that bring the belly muscles into action. This awareness will help to increase your use of belly muscles in each action, and thus tone the muscles all through the day. Also commit to at least five minutes of actual exercising morning and evening, in which you do some of the stress postures I taught you, and then develop your own, a new posture each day of your invention, so that you acquire your own repertoire of movements that you can feel activating your belly muscles.**

Do your best to walk half an hour a day, and run fifteen minutes a day, so that you are activating your warrior spirit regularly.

THE EMOTIONS YOU FEEL. **Make a commitment with your belly that you will regularly pause to see what feelings are being held down there. Breathe into those feelings, and let them come up and** out, rather than being buried in your belly region, where they do nothing but cause trouble for both of you. Each morning, see if you feel like committing to a short session sometime that day in which you get out this book or a guided cassette session and open yourself to emotional release and insight.

THE THOUGHTS YOU THINK. Every day is a new challenge to focus on your self-image, so that your mind can develop a new, stronger and healthier image of how you want your body to look and feel. Talk to yourself about your belly, and visualize how you do look and how you want to look. This is a process that takes quite some time, and in fact is ongoing throughout your lifetime, so develop a regular, conscious habit of encouraging such self-image development. See if you can commit to at least a couple of sessions a week with this book, with a friend, or with a cassette to help you evolve your self-image in positive directions.

⊙

We have looked into your past memories, into your present habits, and into your desired future concerning all four of these primal factors for belly transformation. You now have the tools you need, or know where to get them, and you also have a good, solid understanding of the process of transformation that can enable you to bring your belly into optimum shape and keep it in that shape throughout your life.

But, even more important, I hope you have come to a new relationship with your belly just as it is, so that you can love yourself even in your imperfect condition right now, and let that love be your main vehicle for transforming your belly as the days and weeks and months go by. There is nothing wrong with you right now, and there is nothing keeping you from evolving moment by moment into a new being with a new belly condition— that is the dual magic of life!

So best of luck, love your belly, commit to action, and have a few good belly laughs every day to balance the efforts you make to bring yourself into better shape. Enjoyment of the process is what it is all about!

Supporting
Cassette Programs

As I mentioned earlier, there are times when it is very helpful to put aside the written descriptions of the various programs in this book and to allow yourself to be guided through the exercises, meditations, and reflections by a friendly professional voice on cassette. When you can relax your mind completely, and surrender to the growth process you want to explore, you are able to go much deeper into whatever theme you choose to consider.

In essence, the cassette sessions that accompany this book are modified versions of actual therapy sessions which I use regularly in my practice to guide men toward intimate contact with their bellies. The sessions take for granted that you have read the book already, and they are all aimed at focusing your attention inward, to the various key programs for belly transformation. You can listen to the guided programs many many times, throughout the rest of your life in fact, and each time go deeper into your ongoing relationship with your belly.

BELLY TRANSFORMATIONS: PROGRAM ONE

Side A of this first cassette is a twenty-minute guided session that first takes you into deep present-moment contact with the feelings in your belly, and then guides you back into a number of reflections about your relationship with your belly earlier in your life. There follow a number of verbal affirmations about your desire to improve your belly condition, and several visualization exercises for improving your self-image belly-wise. The session then concludes with five minutes devoted to physical exercises you have learned in the book, which will give your belly muscles a good workout.

Side B, also twenty minutes long, begins with a powerful visualization experience of heroes and warriors you idealized in your childhood and the conditions of their bellies. Then you look back into your own experiences as a child, when you felt a great flow of energy in your body as you imagined yourself a great hero or warrior. You also remember your father's belly and how he treated you power-wise. The session also includes conversations with your belly and additional self-image enhancement exercises. Then eight minutes are devoted to a good physical workout of your belly muscles.

BELLY TRANSFORMATIONS: PROGRAM TWO

Side A is a deep emotional balancing experience in which you explore all twelve of the main emotions that human beings have and bring all of these feelings into a healthy balance within you. By experiencing all these feelings in your belly in one session, you gain an essential sense of integrity in your belly region.

Side B provides you with a specific emotional-release program, so that you can eliminate particular feelings that you find stuck within you while doing the emotional balancing program. This guided emotional-release session is a primary vehicle for awakening the power, vitality, and good feelings in your belly region and in your whole body as well.

BELLY TRANSFORMATIONS: ZEN TUNES

The third cassette is a special musical experience designed to move you through many different emotional and cognitive states. You might want to do your own free-form movements to the music; or you might want to reflect on your relationship with your belly, or any other theme that is dominant in your mind at the time. The music is true meditation music, which, instead of stealing your attention all the time, gives you space within the music for your own inner reflections and meditations. If you consciously breathe deep down in your belly while listening to the different movements of the music, you will find yourself moving effortlessly through the various programs you have learned. In a sense, this third cassette is the advanced, free-form dimension of the belly-transformation programs—as well as simply offering enjoyable relaxing music for whatever you might be doing.

If you would like to order any of these cassettes, you can write to Maurizia Zanin/John Selby Programs, P.O. Box 8320, Santa Fe, New Mexico 87504. $12 per cassette includes postage (check or money order). Your order will be processed and your cassettes mailed within five days, with satisfaction guaranteed.

BELLY TRANSFORMATION SEMINARS

Occasionally I travel around to several cities offering weekend belly-transformation workshops for men wanting to go deeper into their relationship with their bellies and self-image. If you would like information on my workshop schedule, please feel free to write to the above address for the dates and locations near your home. There are also ongoing seminars offered in the Santa Barbara region.

We hope that these cassettes and seminars complement the basic information in the book in ways that further your exploration of that fine belly of yours, and we look forward to your comments and suggestions!